LEADERSHIP
AND ADVOCACY
FOR PHARMACY

LEADERSHIP
AND ADVOCACY
FOR PHARMACY

Edited by

Cynthia J. Boyle

Robert S. Beardsley

David A. Holdford

American Pharmacists Association
Improving medication use. Advancing patient care.
APhA
Washington, D.C.

Editor: Nancy Tarleton Landis
Acquiring Editor: Sandra J. Cannon
Layout and Graphics: Roy Barnhill
Proofreading: Kathleen K. Wolter
Indexing: Suzanne Peake
Cover Design: Richard Muringer

Published by the American Pharmacists Association
1100 15th Street, NW, Suite 400
Washington, DC 20005-1707

To comment on this book via e-mail, send your message to the publisher at
aphabooks@aphanet.org.

Library of Congress Cataloging-in-Publication Data

Leadership and advocacy for pharmacy / Cynthia J. Boyle, Robert S.
Beardsley, and David A. Holdford, editors.
    p. ; cm.
Includes bibliographical references and index.
ISBN-13: 978-1-58212-101-7
ISBN-10: 1-58212-101-X
1. Pharmacy. 2. Leadership. 3. Lobbying. I. Boyle, Cynthia J. II.
Beardsley, Robert S. III. Holdford, David A. IV. American Pharmacists
Association.
[DNLM: 1. Pharmacy. 2. Leadership. 3. Lobbying. 4. Public
Relations. QV 704 L434 2007]
RS122.5.L43 2007
615′.1--dc22
                            2007001664

How to Order This book
Online: www.pharmacist.com
By phone: 800-878-0729 (770-280-0085 from outside the United States)
VISA®, MasterCard®, and American Express® cards accepted

This book is dedicated to our families,
who have taught us important lessons
about leadership and advocacy and
who continue to enrich our lives.

To Martha and Kate

To Kathy, Jessica, and Kyle

To Diane

CONTENTS

PREFACE

The health care professions need effective leadership and, in turn, effective political advocacy to address issues in the complex process of care delivery. Advocacy occurs at many levels, both individual and collective. It can entail the efforts of one pharmacy practitioner on behalf of her patient to improve medication use, or of a group of state pharmacy association officers, pharmacy owners, student pharmacists, or association executives. Publications on leadership theories and development are plentiful, but few are devoted to advocacy. While pharmacists and student pharmacists are asked to be advocates for their profession, they have few opportunities to develop the skills needed for effective advocacy in the political and regulatory arenas. This book articulates, for the next generation of leaders, the value of advocacy skills.

Since effective advocacy cannot occur without effective leadership, this book discusses the elements of effective leadership. Theories related to leadership are presented, along with their application. Rather than simply offering theories or strategies, the book uses the experiences of noted leaders to present lessons that will help pharmacists and student pharmacists become more effective leaders and advocates.

The purpose of this book is threefold: to provide a resource for faculty who teach or desire to teach leadership and advocacy to student pharmacists; to assist students in developing their interests, skills, and abilities to serve as leaders and advocates throughout their careers; and to inspire, inform, and guide practitioners in leadership and advocacy for the profession. The book is offered as a resource for companies, schools, organizations, and health professionals seeking to work with the external environment that legislates and regulates the profession.

The chapters focus on specific aspects of leadership or advocacy as seen from the perspectives of leaders and advocates from a variety of backgrounds. In their chapters and the accompanying personal statements, the authors describe how they became interested in leadership and advocacy, which individuals or events influenced them to become involved, techniques they have found to be most effective, mistakes they have made, and how they have integrated leadership and advocacy into their professional and personal lives.

We would like to thank all the dedicated individuals who contributed to this book. It is our hope, as editors and contributors, that *Leadership and Advocacy for Pharmacy* will benefit the profession.

Cynthia J. Boyle
Robert S. Beardsley
David A. Holdford

February 2007

CONTRIBUTORS

Robert S. Beardsley, RPh, PhD
Professor, Pharmaceutical Health Services Research
School of Pharmacy
University of Maryland
Baltimore, Maryland

Cynthia J. Boyle, PharmD
Director, Experiential Learning Program
Assistant Professor, Pharmacy Practice and Science
School of Pharmacy
University of Maryland
Baltimore, Maryland

Arnold E. Clayman, BS, PD, FASCP
Vice-President, Infusion Services
NeighborCare, an Omnicare Company
Annapolis Junction, Maryland

Ami E. Doshi, PharmD
Student, Class of 2007
Seton Hall University School of Law
Newark, New Jersey

Mary L. Euler, PharmD
Assistant Dean, School of Pharmacy
University of Missouri-Kansas City
Executive Director, Phi Lambda Sigma
Kansas City, Missouri

Joseph Hill, MA
Government Affairs Manager
American Society of Consultant Pharmacists
Alexandria, Virginia

David A. Holdford, BSPharm, MS, PhD
Associate Professor, Pharmacy Administration
School of Pharmacy
Virginia Commonwealth University
Richmond, Virginia

William G. Lang, MPH
Vice President, Policy and Advocacy
American Association of Colleges of Pharmacy
Alexandria, Virginia

Earlene E. Lipowski, PhD
Associate Professor, Pharmacy Health Care Administration
University of Florida
Gainesville, Florida

Raymond C. Love, PharmD, BCPP, FASHP
Vice-Chair, Department of Pharmacy Practice and Science
Director, Mental Health Program
School of Pharmacy
University of Maryland
Baltimore, Maryland

Lucinda L. Maine, PhD
Executive Vice President
American Association of Colleges of Pharmacy
Alexandria, Virginia

John Michael O'Brien, PharmD, MPH
President, Responsible Health, LLC
Bethesda, Maryland

Richard P. Penna, PharmD
Executive Vice President (retired)
American Association of Colleges of Pharmacy
Alexandria, Virginia

Carriann E. Richey, PharmD
Director, Postgraduate Education
Assistant Professor, Pharmacy Practice
College of Pharmacy and Health Sciences
Butler University
Indianapolis, Indiana

Theresa Wells Tolle, BSPharm
Owner, Bay Street Pharmacy and Home Health Care
Sebastian, Florida

Dennis B. Worthen, PhD
Lloyd Scholar, Lloyd Library and Museum
Adjunct Professor, University of Cincinnati College of Pharmacy
Cincinnati, Ohio

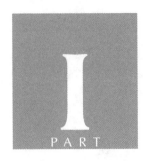

PART

DEVELOPING AND PROMOTING LEADERSHIP

CHAPTER 1

ADVOCACY BY EXAMPLE

Dennis B. Worthen

In the evolution of human endeavors such as the profession of pharmacy, there are important stories to tell. When these stories filter the time-tested from the trivial, they help explain why things are as they are. They tell us what blend of fate and willful deeds of men and women brought us to our current state....

...Many issues relevant to contemporary pharmacists cannot be fully understood without historical perspective. Solutions to many of the problems pharmacy faces may remain elusive without knowing the critical events or trends that shaped them.[1]

The usual definition of a profession comes from the verb "to profess," meaning to claim or declare openly. Advocacy also calls for open declaration on behalf of something or someone else, never in self-interest. There are numerous definitions of leadership, as evidenced by the plethora of self-help books in the management section of any bookstore. The definition of a leader most relevant here, however, is "one who has a commanding influence." Profession, leadership, and advocacy come together in this book about the activities of individuals who want to make something positive happen for pharmacy and pharmacists.

Dennis B. Worthen

Background

Dennis B. Worthen is Lloyd Scholar at the Lloyd Library and Museum in Cincinnati, Ohio. He is also an adjunct professor at the University of Cincinnati College of Pharmacy, where he teaches the history of pharmacy course. He retired from Procter & Gamble Health Care in 1999, after serving as director of pharmacy affairs.

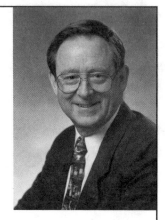

Worthen has authored and edited a number of books on the history of pharmacy, including *Pharmacy in World War II*. He is co-author, with Michael Flannery, of *Pharmaceutical Education in the Queen City: 150 Years of Service 1850–2000*, and he served as editor and author of *The Millis Study Commission on Pharmacy: A Road Map to a Profession's Future*. Worthen was one of the editors of *Reflections on Pharmacy by the Remington Medalists 1919–2003* and is editor-in-chief of the *Dictionary of Pharmacy*. He writes the series "Heroes of Pharmacy" for the *Journal of the American Pharmacists Association*.

Worthen was awarded an Allied Irish Bank Visiting Professorship at the College of Pharmacy at Queen's University in Belfast, Northern Ireland (1986–89). In 1998, he received the Linwood F. Tice Friend of the American Pharmacists Association–Academy of Student Pharmacists Award and the Phi Lambda Sigma National Leadership Award. In 1996 and in 2003, he was the recipient of Fischelis grants from the American Institute of the History of Pharmacy to support his research on pharmacy in World War II. In 2006, he was elected to the International Academy of the History of Pharmacy. Worthen currently serves on the boards of directors of the American Pharmacists Association Foundation and the American Institute of the History of Pharmacy.

From the very beginning of pharmacy in America, there has been a succession of individuals with a vision of what the profession could be, or needed to be, who then served as advocates of that vision to make it reality. Who were these leaders, what were the issues, and why are they still important today? Some may dismiss this inquiry as trivial, dated, or extraneous, but it is not. There have been no advances in American pharmacy that were not the result of individual vision and effort. Advances in educational standards, professional recognition, and societal mission were accomplished by leaders who articulated their vision, advocating it both within the profession and to external audiences, and who made pharmacy what it is today and, equally important, what it will become tomorrow. They succeeded in spite of barriers from outside the profession as well as indifference and apathy within. What are the stories of these leaders and issues, and what is their relevance to today and tomorrow?

Setting Standards

In Philadelphia in 1821, a group of prominent pharmacists came together to form the Philadelphia College of Pharmacy in reaction to the announced plan of the University of Pennsylvania to test and accredit pharmacists. Daniel Smith and the other founders of the college acknowledged that inadequate knowledge and adulterated products were problems for pharmacists; they resolved to effect the necessary changes themselves, rather than be forced to change by another profession. The effort to establish a school for pharmacy apprentices was a struggle—not only with physicians but also with many pharmacists. Physicians complained that the pharmacy teachers were not all that well educated themselves, having merely served an apprenticeship. Some pharmacists were concerned that younger, better-trained practitioners would provide too much competition. But Smith and his colleagues were men of vision who believed that poor pharmacy practice and ignorance of scientific principles must be ended. To pharmacists who feared competition, Smith argued that "we would educate a race of young men better instructed than ourselves, and that if we should be forced by their competition to reform our own shops and to review our old studies, both we and the community would be gainers."[2] Smith was also the force behind the first English-language pharmacy journal in the world. He saw the need for rapid dissemination of new information as an important component of education, not only for members of the Philadelphia college but for all pharmacists.

In response to ongoing problems of imported adulterated products, 20 pharmacists, including Smith and William Procter, Jr., held the organizational meeting of the American Pharmaceutical Association (APhA) in Philadelphia in 1852. This group forged a vision of what pharmacy could be and pledged themselves to work to make it happen. Certainly not representative of pharmacists of that period, they were better educated and predominantly from the organized colleges, all in the East.[3] In preparation for the meeting, Procter wrote about a number of issues, including one that continues to challenge leaders today: How could the new association "hold out inducements sufficient to engage and direct the latent talent of our ranks to such useful and interesting scientific objects as will redound to the improvement of our profession at home, and its reputation abroad?"[4]

Advances in educational standards, professional recognition, and societal mission were accomplished by leaders who articulated their vision, advocating it both within the profession and to external audiences.

A number of individuals envisioned elevating pharmacy education, then little more than a series of evening lectures, to one that equaled the education of other professions. Albert Prescott of the University of Michigan, the founder of the first state university school of pharmacy, broke with the accepted wisdom that students had to have an apprenticeship before attending a college of pharmacy; he instituted laboratory courses as an integral part of what had been totally lecture-based instruction. As a consequence, he was denied a delegate's seat at the 1871 APhA annual meeting, although he was permitted to attend as an individual. Edward Kremers of the University of Wisconsin fought with evangelistic fervor for the place of pharmacy in public education. He introduced the first 4-year university program as an option and argued that the entrance requirements to the university should be the same for pharmacy as for all other programs, since a university education was preparation for lifelong learning: "University courses are to endow men and women with a great capacity for becoming efficient in their calling after they really enter into the same in the every-day battle of life."[5]

One of the most compelling advocates for educational standards was Rufus Lyman, a physician and founding dean of the colleges of pharmacy at the University of Nebraska and, after his retirement, at the University of Arizona. In 1913, when only 1 year of high school was required for admission to a college of pharmacy, Lyman mandated a 4-year high school diploma for admission to the University of Nebraska. It would not be until 1923, however, that this admissions standard was accepted by the American Conference of Pharmaceutical Faculties (now the American Association of Colleges of Pharmacy). As early as 1917, Lyman was at the forefront of the struggle to extend the college course, arguing presciently that the educational standards would not meet the minimum required for government service and that standards needed to be elevated to do justice to all young men and *women* [emphasis added] in pharmacy. The Conference of Faculties initially refused to implement Lyman's expansion, taking the stance that "society" would not stand for it. Lyman continued his drive to extend the college course, first from 2 years to 3 years, and eventually to 4 years. His leadership and advocacy were magnified by his creation of the *American Journal of Pharmaceutical Education* in 1937. Called "Lyman's Journal" by some, the publication was the first English-language publication devoted to pharmacy education. As editor and consulting editor over the next 20 years, Lyman frequently set the agenda for educational standards, advocating education, not training, for future pharmacists.[6]

Securing Roles for Women and Minorities

Two Coopers, Zada Mary and Chauncey, represent inclusion of women and minorities in pharmacy. The two differed in race and gender, but their advocacy for responsibility, excellence, and inclusion was similar. Zada Cooper was a pharmacist and educator when few women were either. She was an outspoken proponent of pharmacists' responsibility to proactively educate the public about self-medication.[7] She served as secretary of the American Association of Colleges of Pharmacy (AACP), the sole paid staff member for 20 years, and frequently joined her friend Rufus Lyman in pressing for higher educational standards. An ardent supporter of women in pharmacy, she maintained that given the opportunity, women would be contributors to society as well as pharmacy. This belief carried over into her founding of Kappa Epsilon. At her retirement from the University of Iowa in 1942, Dean R. A. Kuever remarked that "her influence and service...have made her the most widely known and distinguished woman pharmacist in America today."[8]

Chauncey Cooper was educated at the University of Minnesota College of Pharmacy before accepting a faculty appointment at the first institution established to educate African Americans, Howard University. Few minorities chose pharmacy as a career, and the numbers who did decreased to the point that by 1939 there were fewer than 20 graduates a year. It was a period when many schools of pharmacy refused or restricted minority admission and students had trouble finding employment in stores that would allow them to complete the experiential period necessary for licensure.[9] Invited to write the section on "the Negro in pharmacy" in the Elliott Commission report on the betterment of the profession, Cooper argued for increasing access to pharmacy education, especially in the South, but emphasized that "admission standards should not be relaxed, and a more serious effort should be made to obtain and admit highly competent and well qualified Negro students."[10] Chauncey Cooper was also the founder of the National Pharmaceutical Association, which he envisioned as a means of drawing minorities into the mainstream of American pharmacy.

Gaining Recognition as Professionals

In 1915 Abraham Flexner, author of the well-known report on medical education, refused to do a similar study of pharmacy education, asserting that pharmacy was not a profession, even though its practitioners had special skills that served society. Flexner's position was reflected in the United States military's refusal to recognize pharmacy as a profession. Beginning in 1894, professional associations fought to have pharmacy recognized as a profession in the military. At the heart of the struggle were increased salaries and benefits and officer rank, as well as the question of who should be allowed to prepare medicines (that is, serve as pharmacists) in the military. In 1941 Carl T. Durham, a World War I veteran, pharmacist, and Congressman from North Carolina, was appointed to the House Military Affairs Committee, and in 1942 he introduced a bill titled *To Create a Pharmacy Corps in the United States Army*. General McAfee of the Office of the Army Surgeon General alleged that the role of the pharmacist was technical, simply responding to a physician's order. He stated that most of the medicines used were already in final dose forms and properly labeled so that any "intelligent boy can read the label. And he knows the dangerous ones."[11] It was the persistent, quiet, behind-the-scenes work of Durham that resulted in the passage of the Pharmacy Corps bill in 1943. Durham's advocacy overcame a history of tenacious opposition by 10 Surgeons General of the Army lasting almost 50 years. The Pharmacy Corps itself was superseded by the Medical Service Corps in 1947, but Durham's leadership was evidenced by the fact that all of the armed forces and the Public Health Service recognized pharmacy as a profession and commissioned pharmacists as officers.[12] The Office of Veterans Affairs also recognized pharmacy as a profession. Durham's work as a public servant exemplified the thinking of the executive director of the American Foundation for Pharmaceutical Education, W. Paul Briggs, that "The future place of pharmacy will certainly be a reflection of its value and integrity as a profession, but its comparative status will be determined by its effectiveness on the political stage."[13]

Giving Students a Voice

For more than 100 years after the formation of the first college of pharmacy, students had little voice in the profession. Professional fraternities and sororities started with Phi Delta Chi (1883) and Kappa Epsilon (1921). Rufus Lyman and Zada Cooper were responsible for the establishment of the first pharmacy honor society, Rho Chi, in 1922. In 1965, Auburn University student Charlie Thomas led the formation of Phi Lambda Sigma; the objective of the group was to recognize and promote the leadership efforts of pharmacy students.

Student branches of APhA were authorized with a bylaws change in 1931. By 1953, student branches had been established in most colleges of pharmacy. However, students had minimal presence at the annual APhA meetings and had no voice in policy. Linwood Tice, then dean at the Philadelphia College of Pharmacy, believed that students should be active and have a voice in the Association. At the APhA annual meeting in 1954, the Student

American Pharmaceutical Association was formed; 167 students attended. For the first time, students were represented with a vote in the House of Delegates, giving them an organized voice in the issues and future of their profession. Today the American Pharmacists Association–Academy of Student Pharmacists (APhA-ASP) is one of the organization's three constituent academies.[14]

Tice's belief in student involvement encouraged the creation of a number of quality student-generated programs. Perhaps one of the most enduring examples originated with Marsha Millonig and other students in the University of Minnesota APhA-ASP chapter. They brought the issue of pharmacist impairment to the attention of the state pharmacy association and to the APhA House of Delegates. Although initially unsuccessful, they persisted, and in 1982 the House passed policy supporting the rehabilitation of impaired pharmacists. This student initiative continues through co-sponsorship of the Pharmacy Section of the University of Utah School on Alcoholism and Other Chemical Dependencies.

Moving toward Patient Care

In the mid 20th century it was illegal for pharmacists to counsel patients about their medicines; prescriptions were not labeled for content. Pharmacy students, unlike students in other health professions, had almost no contact with patients; pharmacists were the only health professionals not trained at the patient's bedside. In the 1930s, Edward Spease, dean of the Western Reserve College of Pharmacy, was among the first to articulate the importance of pharmacists training with physicians and nurses. Spease insisted that each of his students have experience in the hospital, but his vision was much broader. He developed standards that required every hospital to have access to graduate pharmacists, something far from common; the American College of Surgeons accepted the standards in 1936. His advocacy resulted in the first graduate degree program in hospital pharmacy. He developed a hitherto unheard of agreement between the hospital and university: that the director of the school and the hospital pharmacy be the same person and that hospital pharmacists have faculty status.[15]

By 1967, Donald Brodie, a faculty member of the University of California–San Francisco, developed the concept of drug-use control, which he defined as a "system of knowledge, understanding, judgment, procedures, skills, controls, and ethics that assures optimum safety in the distribution and use of medication," linking the responsibility of the pharmacist to patient welfare.[16] This was the beginning of what would become clinical pharmacy. In 1973, Brodie first used the term "pharmaceutical care" to describe patient outcomes from the safe use of medicines and a pharmacist's social contract with patients; these efforts to put patient and pharmacist together were a break with the past.[17]

Mary Louise Andersen was a student of Tice at the Philadelphia College of Pharmacy and worked as a community pharmacist for a number of years. In 1974 she joined the Public Health Service, where she worked with migrant and community health programs. Throughout her career Andersen was involved in state and national pharmacy organizations. In 1969 she was elected the first woman speaker of the APhA House of Delegates. She used her leadership position in the federal Health Resources and Services Administration to demonstrate the interdependence between primary health care and pharmaceutical care. Never one to shy away from professional issues, she pressed both government and pharmacy to provide pharmaceutical services to citizens most at risk. Her success in building partnerships to meet the health needs of the underserved was recognized in 2003 when she received the highest professional pharmacy award, the Remington Honor Medal, and in 2004 when the Public Health Service renamed its Nonclinical Pharmacist of the Year Award as the Mary Louise Andersen Leadership Award.

A Continuity of Leaders

Writing in 1950, pharmacy historian George Urdang noted that the profession was fortunate in having a continuity of leaders.[18] From the beginning, when Smith and Procter helped form the first college of pharmacy and the first national professional pharmacy association in the United States, a long succession of individuals have moved pharmacy forward to where it is today. The efforts of

Prescott, Kremers, and Lyman to advance pharmacy education to a university level are evident in today's 6-year, university-based programs. Zada Mary Cooper, Chauncey Cooper, and Tice made inclusion a characteristic of pharmacy; all qualified persons are welcome, regardless of gender or race, and students are an integral part of the profession. Pharmacists in government service today enjoy a professional status that was not possible until Durham's advocacy forced recognition from the military. The shift of emphasis from drug products to the outcomes of therapy for patients, including the patients most at risk, is an ongoing legacy of pharmacists such as Spease, Brodie, and Andersen.

Pharmacy today owes everything to those men and women who had a dream of excellence and the courage to advocate their vision in spite of active barriers and passive indifference. Their examples show that positive change can be made only through individual leadership and advocacy.

In her 2003 Remington address, Andersen described the world as being between the "no longers" and the "not yets," where the old is no longer right even if it is comfortable, and the future is anything but secure. She sounded a clarion call for leaders to be visionaries and advocates for their vision:

> Lead the way, because leaders are called to stand in that lonely place between the "no longers" and the "not yets." We are not called to be popular; we are not called to be safe; and we are not called to follow. We are the ones called to change attitudes and to risk displeasure. We are the ones called to gamble our lives for a better world.[19]

References

1. Zellmer WA. History. In: Zellmer WA. *The Conscience of a Pharmacist: Essays on Vision and Leadership for a Profession.* Bethesda, Md: American Society of Health-System Pharmacists; 2002:178–9.
2. Smith D. Address delivered to the graduates of the Philadelphia College of Pharmacy. *Am J Pharm.* 1837;9:80–98.
3. Worthen DB. Heroes of pharmacy. Founders of the American Pharmaceutical Association. *J Am Pharm Assoc.* 2002;42:892–6.
4. Procter W. Editorial. *Am J Pharm.* 1852;24:186–7.

5. Kremers E. The position of the American Pharmaceutical Association toward pharmaceutical education. *Proc Am Pharm Assoc.* 1895;43:447–53.

6. Worthen DB. Heroes of pharmacy. Rufus Lyman: a towering figure in the field of pharmacy education. *J Am Pharm Assoc.* 2004;44:106–9.

7. Worthen DB. Heroes of pharmacy. Zada Mary Cooper. *J Am Pharm Assoc.* 2003;43:124–6.

8. Kuever RA. Cited in: Coghill MM. Zada Mary Cooper. *The Bond of Kappa Epsilon.* 1965;45(Fall):3–4.

9. Worthen DB. Heroes of pharmacy. Chauncey I. Cooper: champion of minority pharmacists. *J Am Pharm Assoc.* 2006;46:110–3.

10. Cooper CI. The Negro in pharmacy. In: Elliott EC. *The General Report of the Pharmaceutical Survey 1946–1949.* Washington, DC: American Council on Education; 1950:181–7.

11. House of Representatives Committee on Military Affairs, 77th Congress, second session. Hearings on HR 7432, *A Bill to Amend the National Defense Act by Providing for a Pharmacy Corps in the Medical Department, United States Army.* November 17, 1942:8.

12. Worthen DB. Heroes of pharmacy. Carl T. Durham: pharmacy's representative. *J Am Pharm Assoc.* 2005;45:295–8.

13. Briggs WP. Pharmacy must train men in the science of politics. *Am Prof Pharm.* 1962; 28:53–8.

14. Worthen DB. Heroes of pharmacy. Linwood Franklin Tice. *J Am Pharm Assoc.* 2003;43:329–31.

15. Lee CO. Edward Spease. *Am J Pharm Educ.* 1958;22:102–4.

16. Brodie DC. Drug-use control: keystone to pharmaceutical service. *Drug Intell.* 1967;1:63–5.

17. Brodie DC. Is pharmaceutical education prepared to lead its profession? *Report of Rho Chi.* 1973;39(November):6–12. (Ninth Annual Rho Chi Lecture, Boston, July 23, 1973.)

18. Urdang G. The concept of the history of pharmacy. *Am J Pharm Educ.* 1950;14:128–36.

19. Andersen ML. Between the 'No Longer' and the 'Not Yet.' In: Griffenhagen GB, Bowles GC, Penna RP, et al. *Reflections of Pharmacy by the Remington Medalists 1919–2003.* Washington, DC: American Pharmacists Association; 2004:427–31.

Finding Leaders among Us

Lucinda L. Maine

Why Discuss Leadership and Advocacy?

All professions change with time, evolving as those in the profession find new tools and techniques to advance the services they offer to society. It is rare, however, to find examples of professions that have markedly redefined themselves and the work they contribute. Physicians, for example, now have tools that allow them to make more specific diagnoses than in the past, but they still approach medical practice in essentially the same way as their predecessors have for centuries. Teachers have new strategies and technologies to enhance learning, but reading, writing, and math still form the foundation of early childhood education.

Pharmacy is unique in this regard. Parts of our practice have seen changes not unlike those in other professions. For 50 years or more, however, pharmacy's leaders have been working toward a vision of practice significantly different from the way we have operated for much of the 20th century. In a way, pharmacy is making a 360 degree turn, or return, with respect to the provision of direct patient care, but the difference is that the medications and devices now in pharmacists' armamentarium are so much more powerful. Donald E. Francke recognized this more

Lucinda L. Maine

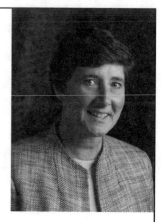

Personal Statement

My earliest recognition that leadership might be in my "gifts portfolio" came in elementary school, when I was tapped as an organizer for such things as the grinder (submarine sandwich) sales that raised funds for our 6th grade class trip to New York City. Sitting on my hands never worked as a deterrent to my natural bent to volunteerism. If there was a job to do, I was one of the first to say yes. My volunteering spirit often led to positions of responsibility and leadership. This continued when I entered pharmacy school at Auburn and soon found myself swept up in the activities of Student APhA (now the American Pharmacists Association–Academy of Student Pharmacists) and Kappa Epsilon.

Many people have influenced my involvement. Student and other pharmacy leaders, on the lookout for rising leadership talent, offered insights into ways to become involved. Advisors, especially Larry Thomasson at Auburn and Al Wertheimer at Minnesota, and deans, like Ben Cooper and Larry Weaver, encouraged me to apply my talents and time to leadership from my earliest days in pharmacy. I was a strong student academically, but they seemed to say "Don't let school interfere with your education; get involved!" Many state and national pharmacy association leaders welcomed me early and throughout my career, and mentored me in ways too numerous to recite.

I think the most important techniques for good leadership relate to communication: listening intently and sincerely to those who wish to make a contribution, and respecting all of those who do. The ability to communicate a vision with optimism has often been cited as a particular strength of mine. Maintaining personal integrity at all costs is also essential.

In terms of mistakes, I think that remaining too insular within pharmacy tops the list. Our future success depends on the help of strong allies from many sources outside the profession, and we spend a bit too much time talking to ourselves. Such internal dialogue may be necessary to create a common vision, but it is insufficient for creating the change we seek in the medication-use process. Other weaknesses in pharmacy leadership may include insufficient organizational acumen to fully operationalize projects and immature delegation skills—a particular weakness early in my career.

As the chief executive officer of a national organization, I call upon leadership and advocacy skills in nearly all I do every day. I find more than a full-time leadership and advocacy challenge in motivating staff to create programs and services that enable academic pharmacy to contribute to quality health care and in communicating with external audiences to help them understand how the changes in pharmacy education serve society by increasing access to medication-use specialists.

than 30 years ago; in his words, "Today's drugs may be likened to ballistic missiles with atomic warheads, while we prescribe, dispense, and administer them as if they were bows and arrows."[1]

As at no time in history, medications and those that help patients manage them have a central role in quality health care.

Leaders are advocates, and engaging in advocacy is an important expectation for many leadership positions.

Examining the history of pharmacy in the United States, we find that pharmacists for many decades provided accessible primary care right on the main square of most towns and cities. Of course, the pharmacists also processed prescriptions written by physicians, but a great deal of their time was spent hearing their patients' health concerns and evaluating whether the nostrums of the day would help alleviate them. As the profession was maturing, pharmacy had little to draw on in terms of patented medicine that actually worked.

The maturation of the medical profession into a powerful political force in society, as well as some twists of state and federal regulations in the mid-1900s, moved pharmacy into an era of subservience. Federal regulations changing the status of medications so that prescription drugs could be dispensed only pursuant to a physician's order, as well as the growing prominence of employed pharmacists as opposed to private entrepreneurs, caused many in the profession to step back as community leaders and activists for change.

Fortunately, leaders such as Donald Brodie, Don and Gloria Francke, William Apple, and Larry Weaver saw pharmacy's future differently. They disliked the subservient roles many pharmacists assumed. Furthermore, these visionaries knew that as medications became more powerful—thanks in large measure to innovative research and development by pharmacists and other researchers in academia and industry—there would be a need for medication-use specialists. They envisioned progressive pharmacy education as the incubator for such expertise. And they could see that this expertise would be needed in every setting where patients receive health care. The thoughts of these giants are captured in numerous papers and study commission reports. The Millis Commission study of pharmacy,[2] published in 1975, is a classic example of the synthesis of the thinking of such visionaries.

State and national pharmacy organizations weighed in, beginning in the 1980s with a series of strategic planning conferences. Leaders in the profession were driven to action by anxiety that pharmacy would not remain a vital player in health care if our future was simply about processing orders for drug products. The vision that pharmacists could make important contributions to quality care by applying their unique medication knowledge and patient care skills was what truly energized the contemporary leaders to plan a course that would complete the return to direct patient care for pharmacists in all settings.

Why Now?

A phenomenon called the "tipping point" has been described by Malcolm Gladwell.[3] If the right leadership is applied to an objective, sometimes the right movement can accelerate when seemingly modest steps are taken. With current attention to problems of health care quality, particularly medication safety and effectiveness, we are at the tipping point for acceptance that the pharmacy profession has two critical functions. As has been true for centuries, we remain responsible for designing and overseeing safe, accurate, and efficient drug distribution systems. Much of the processing of prescriptions today can and should be done by automation and technicians. Leadership and innovation are increasing the opportunities for pharmacists to serve their second key function, as specialists who work with patients and prescribers to design, implement, and monitor medication regimens. It is time pharmacists step up as leaders in health care—as the professionals responsible for providing care that ensures optimal medication therapy outcomes.[4]

The time is right for pharmacy leadership. The work of the Institute of Medicine (IOM) has resulted in the publication of numerous reports on quality and safety in health care. Implementation of health care finance reforms (e.g., pay for performance) and increased scrutiny of the cost, safety, and effectiveness of medications have aligned so that the status quo is no longer acceptable. Either pharmacy as a profession will step forward to lead needed change that improves medication use, or someone else will. Without a doubt, nonpharmacy leadership will not share our vision for the future of our profession.

The most significant consequence of leadership failure and inaction is patient harm. For over a decade, the models of Lyle Bootman and colleagues have suggested that Americans are spending at least as much on the consequences of poorly managed medication use as on medications themselves.[5] Patients suffer unnecessarily; many drug-related problems are predictable consequences of the wrong drug or dose being given, the right drug overlooked, or inadequate monitoring, such as with warfarin therapy.

No one else in the health care system knows as much about the proper use of medications as pharmacists, especially those educated at the doctoral level and with postgraduate residency and other training. The other significant consequence of inaction is that health care leaders will overlook the potential represented by the profession of pharmacy. They will identify other mechanisms for fixing the problems that medication misuse contributes to poor quality care. Pharmacists will be sidelined, their drug distribution roles overtaken by machines and information technology. While this scenario may sound extreme, the profession's leaders have long been motivated by the possibility that it could be our future reality.

Leadership versus Advocacy

Leadership and advocacy are closely related. Leaders are advocates, and engaging in advocacy is an important expectation for many leadership positions. Both leadership and advocacy should be vision-driven. The most effective leaders and advocates are motivated by a cause much bigger than themselves; they should not appear to be seeking recognition for themselves. Integrity is an essential component of leadership and a prerequisite to being an ethical and effective advocate. Finally, leadership and advocacy are needed and applicable at many levels of professional activity and in many different forms.

One difference between leadership and advocacy is their orientation. Advocacy is by design and necessity an externally focused activity; messages are crafted and communicated in order to influence the thinking of a decision-making person or body. Leadership often has both an internal and an external focus; efforts are made to motivate a group to accomplish its goals, and one of the group goals may include advocacy.

Who Me? I'm Not a Leader

Not everyone feels naturally drawn to positions of leadership. Leadership is a gift that some have been given, but, as other authors in this book describe, leadership principles can be learned. Leadership skills can be developed and honed with commitment, opportunity, and dedication. Some people have the false impression that leadership requires assuming a position or gaining a title (e.g., president, chairman, senator), but for the changes that must come to health care to be realized, leadership can and must be developed at many different levels. The most important platform for leadership is in patient care settings, not in the halls of Congress or boardrooms across America. Leading change to improve the quality of medication use requires the leadership of each and every pharmacist in America every day. Contributing to the formation of a functional patient care team is a beautiful example of leading. Advocacy is key to gaining a role for pharmacists on such teams.

It is important that student pharmacists learn from the very beginning to appreciate the need for strong leaders in pharmacy. From first-week orientation sessions to the day of graduation, the dean, faculty, pharmacy preceptors, student organization leaders, and others must stress the critical need for all pharmacy professionals to step up and lead. Student organizations provide wonderful laboratories for leadership development. Participation on committees and leadership in the planning and implementation of events and projects are the building blocks of strong future citizenship. Leadership-building opportunities include working in local communities doing health screenings, working in public schools on literacy projects, and outreach efforts to promote pharmacy careers. Organizing a fundraiser or a social event helps build leadership skills. Participating in a state or national legislative day makes student pharmacists and practicing pharmacists better advocates. Perhaps participation in at least one such activity should be required of every graduating pharmacist before entry into practice.

Leadership and Advocacy and the Pharmacy Curriculum

The Center for the Advancement of Pharmaceutical Education (CAPE) was established by the American Association of Colleges of Pharmacy (AACP) to assist member colleges and schools in their implementation of the Doctor of Pharmacy as the sole professional degree in pharmacy. An important initial contribution of CAPE, in partnership with the profession's practice associations, was identification of the core competencies of pharmacy graduates. These competencies became embedded in pharmacy accreditation standards and drove the development of the Doctor of Pharmacy curriculum at all colleges and schools of pharmacy.

Interestingly, the words "leadership" and "advocacy" do not appear in the CAPE Educational Outcomes for Pharmacy Education updated and published by AACP in 2004.[6] The document focuses instead on where pharmacists should be prepared to apply their knowledge, skills, and abilities in the context of pharmaceutical care, systems management, and public health. That said, each of these arenas of practice is a target for strong pharmacy leadership and advocacy for quality improvement. A few words about each of these three overarching areas of competency will illustrate.

The delivery of pharmaceutical care services in all health care settings draws upon the leadership and advocacy skills of pharmacists in numerous ways, as such services are still novel and innovative in far too many practices today. Practice leaders must first have a vision that this is the level of service that must be available to patients. Leaders must be able to communicate that effectively to others with authority, especially to the other health care providers with whom the pharmacists will collaborate. It is essential that pharmacy education equip graduates not just with the knowledge of medications and their proper use, but also with the vision and skills to be agents of change.

The 2004 CAPE outcomes with regard to systems management are the least novel yet the least developed aspect of contemporary pharmacy curricula. Ensuring that safe, accurate, and efficient drug distribution systems operate within our practices has always been a core function of pharmacy. What has changed today is the complexity of such systems. With new technology and sophisticated drug therapy, a great deal of leadership is needed to design, operate, and evaluate drug-use management systems in all settings of care. Perhaps most important in this component of the curriculum are the knowledge and skills related to quality improvement and the effective use of informatics in health care. These are two of the five core competencies in the IOM report on health professions education.[7] Pharmacy education and practice needs a substantial amount of leadership and involvement in interprofessional efforts to incorporate quality measurement and accountability into the delivery of care. The appropriate use of information systems to enhance quality care similarly requires substantial leadership, both in health care settings and at broader policy levels within the public and private sectors.

Within the third area of competency in the CAPE outline, public health and prevention, is the subcompetency "develop health policy." Without question, this competency is about leadership and advocacy, and the profession must give priority to expanding the number of individuals prepared and motivated to contribute to the development of informed health policy. If we fail to do so, others with less insight into the safe and effective management of pharmaceuticals as a central component of health care will be making the decisions in delineating health policy.

An example of policy and public health leadership in pharmacy at the local, state, and national levels is in the area of immunization advocacy and delivery. In the early 1990s, government officials at all levels up through the White House realized that the United States had fallen far short of goals to have its citizens appropriately immunized. Pharmacy leaders recognized an opportunity to make the case that pharmacists could play an important role in helping the country meet its immunization goals. Focused advocacy efforts changed state laws and regulations to secure immunization authority in virtually every state.

This required negotiation with public health officials and the medical and nursing leaders in the states. Ultimately, it required the passionate vision of pharmacy leaders who relentlessly pursued a goal of adding the value of pharmacists' location, education, and patient relationships to the quest to properly immunize those vulnerable to vaccine-preventable disease.

These are but a few examples of the ways in which leadership skills contribute to advancing pharmacy practice at the local, state, and national level. Stimulating student pharmacists and practitioners to recognize and fully develop those skills is an essential responsibility of the colleges and schools of pharmacy.

Importance of Partnerships

The phrase "TEAM stands for Together Everyone Achieves More" rings so true. All who share the vision for improving health care must work collaboratively on solutions that will increase access to quality care for everyone in society. Significant leadership can and should come from colleges and schools of pharmacy, but not in isolation from a wide array of partners. Practicing pharmacists, pharmacy educators, corporate and association leaders, and those in other health care disciplines are all allies in the quest for quality in health care.

An excellent example of a partnership opportunity exists in the experiential component of pharmacy education today. Only a small portion of advanced practice rotations are directed and supervised by full-time pharmacy faculty. Clinical education represents approximately 25% to 30% of pharmacy students' education—a significant component. The need to build a cadre of adjunct faculty members and equip them with the knowledge and materials they need to serve as advanced practice preceptors is a marvelous opportunity for pharmacy education to partner with the practice community.

In addition, pharmacy educators have consistently served as pioneers in bringing pharmaceutical care services to a variety of health care settings. There are many examples of collaboration between schools of pharmacy and hospitals, clinics, and pharmacies in the community that have resulted in innovative patient care practices and rotation sites. Such partnerships must be built on a shared vision for fully utilizing the knowledge and skills of pharmacy practitioners to deliver quality, patient-focused care. Pharmacy faculty can serve as role models and mentors for practitioners and help organize and deliver innovative services. Faculty and students can reach out to physicians and others in the community or institution to identify their needs for better medication management services by pharmacists. In such partnering, everyone wins; the practice expands its service dimensions, students have excellent learning opportunities, and patient care is improved.

Leaders in medical education and other health disciplines have watched with great interest the transformation in pharmacy education with the move to the professional doctoral degree. Over decades, many other health professions educators have come to appreciate the contributions pharmacists and student pharmacists make to patient care in hospitals, and slowly it is dawning on these academic leaders that medications also play a key role in patient management in ambulatory settings. Building upon this recognition to strengthen partnerships in interprofessional education and practice is a high priority of AACP and its members. Team-delivered care is better patient care and is the vision of the future for leaders from all health care disciplines, including pharmacy.

Expectations of Practitioners, Students, Faculty, and Organizations

Health care is targeted for change from many directions. Politicians, business leaders, insurers, patient advocacy groups, and health professions themselves are committed to the redesign of health care financing and delivery to create a system that is safer, more patient-focused, and affordable for all. This is a tall order, one that cannot be accomplished successfully without a substantial amount of leadership from the pharmacy profession.

As noted throughout this book, there are innumerable ways to provide leadership, and all are needed and important. Connections at the community level afford pharmacists and student pharmacists opportunities to broaden others' thinking about the full range of contributions pharmacists make to society. One can never be sure how the comments made at a Rotary meeting or at the board meeting of a local free clinic might influence others to engage and support pharmacy in new and different ways.

Student pharmacists, through the organizations established at each pharmacy school, have numerous channels for outreach, service, and leadership development. Volunteering for a committee, coordinating an event, seeking an elected position, speaking up, and being engaged are all essential components of professionalism and should possibly even be requirements for completing a degree in pharmacy. Local, state, and national pharmacy organizations also need the active support of students as well as practitioners. There is, unfortunately, too much "freeloading" in our profession. Assuming that others will carry the mantle of leadership is nothing short of a cop-out—an abrogation of a practitioner's professional duty. Inactive pharmacists have no one but themselves to blame if pharmacy loses ground in the mind of the public or in the public policy arena.

How Do We Measure Success or Effectiveness?

One reason that pharmacists and others may be reluctant to actively engage in leadership and advocacy efforts is that it can be difficult to see tangible and immediate results. What does one telephone call to a member of Congress yield? Can a single health screening led by student pharmacists and faculty really make a difference? It is a rare event, especially at the federal level, to actually see advocacy efforts translated into something as concrete as a piece of legislation passed by both the House and the Senate and signed into law by the President.

Despite the often amorphous character of advocacy and leadership work, it is important to keep several things clearly in mind. The profession's leaders share a vision for what pharmacists can and will contribute to society. As long as our individual or group advocacy and leadership efforts contribute in ways small or large to that shared vision, those contributing can consider their work to be effective.

However, each initiative should have clear objectives, even if it is as simple as an effort to mobilize student pharmacists to send e-mail or letters to the state legislature or board of pharmacy to draw attention to a regulation that prevents pharmacists or students from realizing their full potential. Certainly, a change in the regulation is the outcome desired eventually, but mobilizing dozens of communications clearly stating the case should be considered a positive intermediate outcome.

Margaret Mead has been quoted as saying, "Never doubt that a small group of thoughtful, committed citizens can change the world; indeed, it's the only thing that ever has." This is our call to action and the promise that our efforts will, indeed, make a difference in the quality of health care our patients receive.

References

1. American Pharmaceutical Association. *The Role of the Pharmacist in Comprehensive Medication Use Management: The Delivery of Pharmaceutical Care* [position paper]. Washington, DC: American Pharmaceutical Association; March 1992.
2. American Association of Colleges of Pharmacy. *Pharmacists for the Future: The Report of the Study Commission on Pharmacy.* Ann Arbor, Mich: Health Administration Press; 1975.
3. Gladwell M. *The Tipping Point: How Little Things Can Make a Big Difference.* Boston: Back Bay Publishing; 2002.
4. Joint Commission of Pharmacy Practitioners. *JCPP Future Vision of Pharmacy Practice.* Available at: www.aacp.org/site/pdf.asp?TP=/Docs/Main Navigation/Resources/6725_JCPPFutureVisionofPharmacyPractice FINAL.pdf. Accessed December 15, 2006.
5. Johnson J, Bootman JL. Drug-related morbidity and mortality: a cost-of-illness model. *Arch Intern Med.* 1995;155:1949–56.
6. American Association of Colleges of Pharmacy. CAPE Educational Outcomes 2004. Alexandria, Va: American Association of Colleges of Pharmacy; 2004.
7. Institute of Medicine. *Health Professions Education: A Bridge to Quality.* Greiner AC, Knebel E, eds. Washington, DC: National Academies Press; 2003.

CHAPTER

Leadership Theories for Leading Change

David A. Holdford

I f you thought you could make a change in the pharmacy profession, would you be willing to try? If you had the leadership skills and qualities to effectively promote the professional image of pharmacists and increase their influence within the health care system, would you use them? If you had the power to change things, would you do so? Most of us would probably say yes to these questions, because we see things that need to be improved in our profession. This chapter is designed to show you how to lead change.

Across the country, pharmacists and students like you are making a difference in our profession. This book offers examples of leaders who are passionate about their chosen causes and are using their leadership skills to advocate and influence change. What sets them apart from nonleaders is that they care enough to work for change.

Phases of Leadership Growth

The typical pharmacist does not graduate with extensive leadership capabilities. I consider myself a typical pharmacist—I'm

David A. Holdford

Background

David A. Holdford is Associate Professor, Pharmacy Administration, at Virginia Commonwealth University (VCU; Medical College of Virginia Campus) School of Pharmacy in Richmond. He completed his BS in Pharmacy at University of Illinois, Chicago; MS in Pharmacy Administration at Ohio State University; and PhD in Pharmacy Administration at University of South Carolina. Before joining the VCU faculty in 1995, Holdford worked as a pharmacist and manager at hospitals in Chicago and Columbia, South Carolina. At VCU, he teaches professional and graduate students about pharmacist leadership, the marketing of pharmaceuticals and pharmacist services, and other topics important to contemporary pharmacy practice. Holdford's current research interests focus on pharmacoeconomics, health outcomes assessment, and the role of marketing in health care. He has published more than 50 articles and book chapters in health care and business publications and is the author of the textbook *Marketing for Pharmacists,* published by the American Pharmaceutical Association.

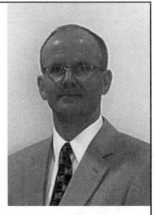

Holdford describes in this chapter his own road to leadership.

relatively intelligent, I work hard, and I care about others. My grades were good in pharmacy school, and I even completed a graduate degree, taking courses in organizational behavior, psychology, and sociology to better understand people and their behaviors. After graduation, I worked for 5 years as a hospital pharmacist. Observing others in leadership positions caused me to conclude, "I can do a lot better than that." I assumed that I was ready for success as a pharmacist manager, but I was wrong.

I was unprepared for the demands of being a manager. My education and training really did not help me understand how to manage and lead others. I naively thought that my managerial title gave me power over the people I supervised, but they regularly resisted my ideas and proposals. The resistance was rarely overt. Instead, opposition usually took the form of a lack of commitment to the things I felt were important. Although co-workers might go through the motions of accepting my initiatives, they usually exerted minimal effort toward making them succeed.

It was surprising to learn that many of the managerial dilemmas I faced were not easily solved by common sense or textbook solutions. For instance, it was very difficult for me to balance the competing demands of my employer, boss, and co-workers with my personal desires and family responsibilities. Someone always seemed to be unhappy, and it made me feel bad. My problems were compounded by the fact that the skills and behaviors that made me a successful staff pharmacist did not necessarily make me a good manager. Sadly, I failed as a manager and leader more often than I really want to admit—initially. But as my career progressed, I learned from my mistakes and began to succeed as a leader.

My leadership training progressed through four different phases of growth described by Maxwell.[1] The first was "I don't know what I don't know." In this phase, I did not realize my deficiencies as an effective leader. I had an inflated sense of my capabilities and contributions to the pharmacy. When problems occurred, I was more likely to blame my boss or co-workers than to assume any responsibility for a problem. Over time, however, I moved to the second phase of leadership growth, "I now know what I don't know." At this point, it began to dawn on me that my own inexperience and ignorance were the reason for many of my failures as a manager. It became clear that I did not have the answer to all problems and that my success hinged upon the people with whom I worked. It was also apparent that many of the assumptions I made about leadership were incorrect and that my behavior needed to change if I wanted to gain the respect and trust of those I managed. It was in this second phase that I dedicated myself to becoming a student of leadership and learning what it takes to become a leader. I observed leaders in my life and in the public arena and reflected on what caused them to succeed or fail. I read a lot of leadership books, too.

Nevertheless, it was not until the third phase, "I now know and it is starting to show," that I truly began to develop as a leader. In this third phase, I applied what I'd learned about leadership to my work and everyday personal life. I identified personal weaknesses and bad habits that were holding me back as a leader and systematically worked to improve upon them. For example, I sometimes carelessly forgot about the promises I'd made to others. This would lead them to conclude that I didn't care about them or their feelings, and it hurt my credibility with them. To correct this bad habit and repair my relationships with co-workers, I developed a habit of noting each of my promises in a pocket calendar, along with a deadline for responding to the person to whom I'd made the promise. This helped me remember my promise and reminded me when I failed to keep it. Then, if I forgot a promise, I was clearly aware of it, making me more determined to keep my word in the future. By systematically identifying and changing similar ineffective behaviors, I developed better personal and professional relationships and increased my leadership effectiveness. Furthermore, I sought out additional opportunities to develop my skills by choosing different tasks that stretched my capabilities. Rather than seeing these tasks as additional work, I viewed them as leadership training. Over time, I grew as a leader and my effectiveness became noticeable to others. It was when others recognized me as a leader that I realized I truly was one.

I now find myself in the final leadership growth phase, "I now lead because it is what I am." In this phase, leadership is no longer a conscious act; it is just a part of my life. That is not to say that I don't make mistakes or that I don't have a lot more to learn about leading. It just means that I've reached a point where I am not consciously aware when I influence others. I just do it, because it is a natural extension of what I am and what I want to achieve. I still consciously assess my leadership performance and adjust my behavior accordingly. However, many of my leadership behaviors have been internalized and become a part of me.

The Need for Different Leadership Styles

Some of the difficulties I faced in my first formal managerial position occurred because I used the wrong leadership approach for the circumstances. I tried to use a democratic leadership approach, as I had in my previous staff pharmacist position. However, I found that democratic leadership is not effective in every situation. Indeed, I discovered that no single leadership style can be effective in all situations because leadership conditions differ and constantly change. Effective leaders must recognize and adapt to the changing circumstances. A leader's ability to adapt will grow as he or she masters and effectively uses different approaches.

Six approaches to leadership are discussed in the following paragraphs: coercive, affiliative, transformational, democratic, pacesetting, and coaching (Table 3-1).[2]

Coercive. The coercive leadership style relies on the use of rewards and punishments to motivate followers. It can be very effective in getting people to take action but can be seen as manipulative and demeaning. A leader who dangles rewards in front of followers or threatens to punish them essentially says, "Do this or else." This style might get people to act, but they will likely do so with little enthusiasm. It emphasizes the leader's power over followers and generates an adversarial relationship of "us versus them." Coercion can hurt relationships with followers, especially highly productive ones, because it does not treat them as mature, contributing individuals. To the contrary, coercion undermines pride in mature adults and encourages passivity by teaching them to wait for incentives from the leader before acting. Coercion is also ineffective when leaders have little ability to reward or punish, such as when working with volunteers or when followers are more intrinsically motivated by the work in which they engage than by the extrinsic rewards received for completing that work.

Hence, coercive leadership is best used sparingly. It should be reserved for crisis situations in which quick and firm action is required. It may also be used temporarily in support of other leadership styles. For example, a co-worker who does not keep a promise may be told, "I feel as though you let us down. You did not do what you promised. We need to know that we can rely on you in the future. Your help is critical to our success." Within this statement is an implied threat that behavior must improve or something will happen. At the same time, the statement supportively emphasizes the co-worker's importance. Nevertheless, coercion is not desirable over the long term in most leadership situations. It is better to use one of the other five styles of leadership whenever possible.

Affiliative. The affiliative style of leadership revolves around meeting the emotional needs of followers. It focuses on people, whereas coercive leadership focuses on the task. Affiliative leaders seek happiness, harmony, and, ultimately, loyalty between

TABLE 3-1   Comparison of Leadership Styles

Style	Description	Advantages	Disadvantages
Coercive	Relies on rewards and punishments to influence followers.	Can influence behavior quickly if rewards are valued or punishments feared.	May be seen as manipulative and result in resentment. Once rewards and punishments are gone, effort can diminish. Not all leaders have coercive authority or resources.
Affiliative	Provides support for the emotional needs of followers.	Encourages communication, belonging, teamwork, trust, independence, and satisfaction.	An overemphasis on individual needs of followers may occur at the cost of organizational performance.
Transformational	Inspires others through a shared vision of the future.	When followers share the same vision as leaders, they are highly motivated and need little further direction.	Visions must be continually reinforced so followers are not distracted and the vision remains clear. The credibility of leaders must also be maintained.
Democratic	Provides each person with equal say in decisions.	Attains buy-in and commitment from followers by demonstrating respect. Encourages followers to take responsibility for their work and work outcomes.	Can be painfully inefficient. Requires rules of conduct that are explicit and accepted by both followers and leaders.
Pacesetting	Leads by example.	Powerfully demonstrates high expectations of the leader through actions. Pacesetters can gain credibility with followers this way.	Expectations set by example but not words can be ambiguous and hard to pin down. Guidelines for acceptable performance are not explicit if they are based only on actions. Followers are left to guess what the leader wants.
Coaching	Encourages self-development and motivation by helping followers develop themselves according to their personal and career aspirations.	Empowers followers to act independently. Challenges them to improve. Tries to link goals of organization to goals of followers.	Takes significant time and effort up front for the leader. Requires patience from the leader and a willingness to let followers fail as they learn.

leaders and followers. They use communication and trust-building activities to develop relationships. They share ideas and concerns with followers and encourage them to do the same. Affiliative leaders emphasize positive feedback for good work in order to build up confidence and self-esteem. When criticism is offered, it is provided with the greatest care and concern for an individual's feelings. Affiliative leaders try to build a strong sense of inclusion and teamwork.

Affiliative leadership is effective as long as leaders do not ignore the task at hand. Group inclusion and loyalty should never be the goal, but only a means of achieving the organization's goal. If group harmony is nurtured at the expense of good performance, neither the organization nor individuals are well served.

Transformational. Transformational leaders direct followers toward a shared vision of the future. They transform the leader's vision into one that can be shared by followers; this is often seen as the purest form of leadership.[3] Transformational leaders use their vision to inspire others with dreams of what can be. Martin Luther King, Jr., Ronald Reagan, and Mother Teresa can all be considered transformational leaders who inspired others through actions and words. Each had an inspiring vision of the future that was adopted by followers.

Transformational leadership frequently succeeds because it is highly motivating. Transformational leaders communicate to followers how their work fits into a shared vision, and then let followers choose and implement strategies for achieving the vision. This responsibility can empower followers and is flexible enough to permit imaginative solutions to problems.

The success of transformational leadership lies in the leader's ability to communicate a clear and lasting vision to followers. Once established, the vision must be continually reinforced lest followers lose their direction. If it is not reinforced, competing messages and changing circumstances can diminish the power of a vision. The transformational leader must also avoid losing credibility in the eyes of followers, because their commitment to the vision is commonly founded on trust in the leader. Consequently, the leader's personal character and ability to communicate are important for successful transformational leadership.

Democratic.   Democratic leaders solicit input from followers and attain their buy-in for major decisions and initiatives. Participative democracy shows respect to followers and helps build their commitment more effectively than simply telling them what to do. Encouraging their input can also provide a broader range of solutions and push followers to take greater responsibility for their success. Morale increases, too, because followers feel valued and part of the change process.

The primary drawback of democracy is that it can be frustratingly inefficient. It typically results in too many meetings, debates, and negotiations. Reaching consensus also leads to compromises that produce less than optimal results, especially when deadlines are to be met. On the other hand, democracy can bring many minds to bear on a problem and lead to group commitment to a plan of action. In truth, group commitment to a mediocre plan is usually preferred to weak backing of the best plan. The key to successful democratic leadership is to establish and enforce an explicit and accepted process for the conduct of all individuals (e.g., bylaws, policies, and procedures). Accepted rules for behavior help ensure an orderly democratic process.

Pacesetting.   Pacesetting occurs when leaders demonstrate expected behaviors through their own personal actions. Commonly called leading by example, this is considered an admirable form of leadership. In essence, the leader says, "Do as I do." This is the type of leadership seen in military officers who lead the charge or star athletes who lead the team. Pacesetters often gain credibility with followers by setting a good example.

A major problem with pacesetting can be that it sends unclear messages about desired performance.[2] The meanings of a leader's actions can be ambiguous. For instance, a pacesetter may want to communicate through his actions the message, "If we all work hard, we will succeed." But the follower may interpret the leader's message as, "If you do not work as hard as I do, you aren't good enough." Or, the actions of pacesetters may be misinterpreted as an expectation of conformity by followers, devaluing their individuality. With pacesetting as the primary style, no one can ever be as good as the leader, who is the "gold standard." Furthermore, followers often have to guess the leader's intentions because expectations of performance are typically locked away in the leader's mind. Ambiguity about what is expected can cause anxiety and low morale in followers. It is similar to being given tests in college and never knowing if the answers are correct or what scores are needed to pass.

Effective leadership is needed to help pharmacists organize and coordinate their advocacy efforts.

Still, leading by example is a very useful style. It is most effective for managing teams of highly motivated and self-directed individuals, such as medical teams in a hospital or professional sports teams.[2] It also works well when used in combination with other styles that supplement the pacesetter's actions with explicit written and spoken communication. Actions may speak louder than words, but words clarify the meanings of those actions.

Coaching. The coaching style encourages followers to develop their skills and capabilities, with the goal of improving performance and increasing their ability to take on greater responsibilities. The goal of coaching is to develop followers so that they no longer need assistance from leaders. Followers are encouraged to identify personal goals that match those of the leader and organization. Subsequently, the coach and follower collaboratively establish long-term plans to meet their mutual needs. For instance, the president of a student organization may direct a member to volunteer for an open position as chair of a subcommittee, if that member aspires to run for future office. When the new subcommittee chair succeeds, everyone benefits.

Coaching's biggest drawback is the time and patience it requires. It is often easier in the short run to do something yourself or just tell someone what to do. It also takes substantial patience and self-control for leaders to share responsibility and be tolerant of mistakes as followers learn new tasks and skills. In the long run, however, well-coached individuals rarely need to be told what to do, and they share the workload with leaders. Coaching leadership benefits organizations by growing future leaders. It also builds commitment by telling followers, "I believe in you and your potential enough to invest my time with you. I know that you will succeed." This powerful message is typically met by the best efforts of followers.

Using Multiple Leadership Styles

Effective leaders use a broad range of leadership styles to encourage others to advocate change. At Virginia Commonwealth University, pharmacy students have been active in school governance, holding various leadership roles in student, school, and local organizations. One student leader (DK) succeeded in seamlessly switching from one style to another depending on the specific situation. DK was transformational because he identified and articulated a clear, persuasive vision for what he wanted to achieve at the school. One element of his vision was that students who adopt professional behaviors in pharmacy school will be more professional as pharmacists. DK argued that a code of student behavior and dress should be adopted for all students. Although this viewpoint was not universally accepted by his classmates, his vision was moved forward by students who did share his viewpoint. Another element of DK's vision was that good leaders prepare others for leadership. Thus, he helped coach other students to be better leaders. His credibility was such that he could provide feedback in a manner that was appreciated and valued by others. It helped that DK never let his ego get in the way; he shared credit with others, and he always listened to and respected others' viewpoints. He democratically let the majority rule even when he did not agree with the decision. And once a decision was made, he did not second-guess it or complain. His inclusive and nonjudgmental manner made everyone around him feel good. He worked hard and set a good example for others, but he never used pacesetting as a vehicle for self-aggrandizement or sympathy. He never mentioned his own efforts, preferring to highlight the efforts of others. His use of pacesetting was effective because it was done quietly, without strong expectations of others. Indeed, his efforts were inspirational because they emphasized his commitment to his vision. There were few students or faculty members who did not know and respect him.

Although the management literature provides some guidance on appropriate leadership styles in changing situations, the ultimate determinant of good leadership is the ability to achieve your goals. Theories can only inform your behaviors. It takes application and experience to identify a blend of styles that works best for you.

You Can Lead and Not Be in Charge

Some people think they must possess a formal leadership position in order to lead change. On the contrary, anyone can lead. In my first job as a hospital pharmacist in Chicago during the 1980s, I worked with a pharmacy technician who was nicknamed "IR." IR was a pharmacist from India who took a job at the hospital as a technician until he could meet the requirements for the Illinois pharmacist licensing exam. Officially, I was his superior and responsible for supervising his work, but in reality, his influence on the day-to-day work in the pharmacy was much greater than mine. Although a technician, IR never let his official role limit his influence on how pharmacy was practiced at the hospital. He developed credibility as someone who could be relied upon in any situation, and he used that credibility to suggest ways to improve our patient care. He typically took the lead in implementing new ideas.

IR realized that his ability to influence was not limited by his formal position. He understood that the power to influence can come from different sources:

- **Formal power** is awarded to individuals when they accept some position of formal authority, such as an office in a student organization or a position as a pharmacy manager. As a technician, IR had little formal authority because he had no official authorization to reward or punish, make budgetary decisions, or set policy. Instead, he wielded other, nonformal powers.
- **Reward power** refers to one's ability to reward others who act in a desired manner. Although this is often associated with formal positions of authority, anyone can reward others. IR rewarded people by helping out whenever needed, providing encouraging words, showing that he cared for them, and making work more fun.

- **Punishment power,** the converse of reward power, exists in a person's ability to punish. This, too, is not restricted to formal positions of authority. IR rarely used this form of power, although he could easily have punished co-workers with an unkind word or a dirty look. He avoided the use of punishments, because he believed they damaged personal relationships and were thus counterproductive as a means of influencing change.

- **Expert power** is derived from a person's special knowledge, skills, and experience. Influence comes when others rely on that person's expertise. IR developed expertise through his knowledge of policies and technical aspects of running the pharmacy. Consequently, he was regularly consulted about issues of importance to running the pharmacy.

- **Information power** derives from the possession of critical information needed by others. Beyond his expertise, IR often possessed unique information because he developed strong relationships with technicians, pharmacists, and managers. His professionalism, pleasant demeanor, and competence gave others the confidence to share information with him.

- **Referent power** is an individual's ability to influence another by force of character or charisma. IR's referent power came from the goodwill and mutual respect he built over time with others in the pharmacy.

I learned from IR that anyone can be a leader if he or she so desires. Although IR was a technician, he developed considerable power in the pharmacy to influence practice. IR would probably deny his leadership role, but he was clearly recognized as a leader among his peers. All of us can be leaders whenever we choose to take a stand and act to influence others. We must realize that we should never be limited by our formal titles.

A major step in leading change is to understand the power you possess and are willing to use. If you want to start leading, you should identify a situation at work, school, or home where you desire some change. Then, think about the different sources of power you have to influence the situation. You will probably be surprised to learn that you possess more power than you originally thought. As you exert your power, you will progress as a leader.

How to Develop Leadership Capabilities

Seek to better understand yourself. When learning to lead, you must assess your current capabilities and identify the skills you need to develop. The more you know about what motivates you, how your emotions affect your reactions to circumstances, what your personal strengths and weaknesses are, and what you want to achieve as a leader, the better. Self-assessment can be conducted through formal tests (e.g., Myers-Briggs Type Indicator) and through the feedback of friends, family, employers, and co-workers. This self-knowledge is useful in developing skills as a leader and learning to adapt to leadership demands.

Learn about leadership from others. Leadership training can be facilitated through observation. Students of leadership identify leaders and observe how they influence others. They examine leaders in their personal lives, and by reading about them in the news and reading their books, and then reflect on what works and does not work for them. Students of leadership observe which leadership styles are best employed in different situations, how followers respond to the different styles, and how things might have been done differently. Identifying and working with a mentor during your early stages of leadership growth can facilitate this process.

Practice leadership yourself. Leadership is a performing art, mastered only through participation and practice. Reading about leadership and observing others may help, but true mastery does not happen until you are faced with the tough decisions of leading. Look for opportunities to lead at work, school, home, and almost anywhere people interact. Simply choose a cause about which you are passionate and then take the leap. Your passion can be about something small (e.g., littering) or very large (e.g., world peace). With experience and time, you will move from "I don't know what I don't know" to "I now lead because it is what I am."

Conclusion

No pharmacist, acting alone, can be an effective advocate for the profession. Change can occur only when pharmacists act together. Effective leadership is needed to help pharmacists organize and coordinate their advocacy efforts. Pharmacists who understand and apply basic leadership principles can multiply their ability to advocate for change in the profession. Effective leaders strengthen advocacy efforts by energizing others to work with them and inspiring them to work toward a shared vision of the future.

The need for leadership in the pharmacy profession is well recognized in the literature.[4-7] A concern often expressed is that too few pharmacists have the training and experience needed to succeed in leading the profession. Our hope is that the stories presented in this book will inspire you to use your power for positive change.

References

1. Maxwell JC. *The 21 Irrefutable Laws of Leadership.* 1st ed. Nashville, Tenn: Thomas Nelson, Inc; 1998.
2. Goleman D. Leadership that gets results. *Harvard Bus Rev.* March-April 2000:78–90.
3. Kotter JP. What leaders really do. *Harvard Bus Rev.* May-June 1990:103–11.
4. Engle JP. Leadership and professionalism in pharmacy. *Am J Health Syst Pharm.* 1991;48:1559–62.
5. Maine LL. Leadership in pharmacy. *Am J Health Syst Pharm.* 1988; 45:2537–41.
6. Manasse HR. The power of pharmacy leadership. *Am J Health Syst Pharm.* 2005;62:1700–2.
7. Holdford DA. Leadership theories and their lessons for pharmacists. *Am J Health Syst Pharm.* 2003;60:1780–6.

Additional Resources

Phi Lambda Sigma, The National Pharmacy Leadership Society (www. philambdasigma.org)

The American Society of Health-System Pharmacists has leadership resources on its Web site (www.ashp.org/).

The *Harvard Business Review* has excellent articles on leadership and related topics (harvardbusinessonline.hbsp.harvard.edu).

Abrashoff M. *It's Your Ship: Management Techniques from the Best Damn Ship in the Navy.* New York: Warner Business Books; 2002. This book by a retired U.S. Navy Captain illustrates how multiple leadership styles were used in command of the destroyer *USS Benfold*.

Covey S. *The 7 Habits of Highly Effective People.* New York: Free Press; 2004. Habits for success.

Maxwell JC. *The 21 Irrefutable Laws of Leadership.* Nashville: Nelson Business; 1998. This is the best of a series of books by Maxwell on leadership.

Thomas KW. *Intrinsic Motivation at Work—Building Energy and Commitment.* San Francisco: Berrett-Koehler; 2002. Good discussion of how to motivate yourself and others.

STUDENT LEADERSHIP DEVELOPMENT

Ami E. Doshi

> Here's to the crazy ones. The misfits. The rebels. The troublemakers. The round pegs in the square holes. The ones who see things differently. They're not fond of rules, and they have no respect for the status quo. You can quote them, disagree with them, glorify or vilify them. About the only thing that you can't do is ignore them. Because they change things....They push the human race forward....While some may see them as the crazy ones, we see genius. Because the people who are crazy enough to think they can change the world are the ones who do.

> —"Think Differently," Apple Computer advertisement

Student pharmacists are the future of the pharmacy profession. Some are even crazy enough to think they can change the world. Many see the big picture more clearly than some practitioners can—these are the upcoming leaders of the profession. Most students do not enter pharmacy school as born health care leaders, however. Their value systems, morals, and ethics have developed before they enter pharmacy school, but their educational journey presents them with issues that challenge their integrity and shape the application of their principles.

Ami E. Doshi

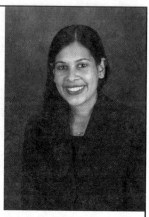

Background

Ami E. Doshi graduated with honors from the Ernest Mario School of Pharmacy at Rutgers University in 2004. During pharmacy school, she was actively involved in the American Pharmacists Association–Academy of Student Pharmacists (APhA-ASP) and the New Jersey Pharmacists Association (NJPhA). These activities provided Doshi with opportunities to serve on national committees and meet students and practitioners from different areas of the country and, during her last year of school, she served as National Speaker of the APhA-ASP House of Delegates.

By the end of her pharmacy education, Doshi had decided to go to law school; she enrolled in Seton Hall Law School as a Distinguished Scholar in Health Law. Now in her third and final year of school, she works in community pharmacy and continues to be an active member of APhA and NJPhA. Currently, she is symposium editor of the *Seton Hall Law Review* and president of the Health Law Forum. Working as a summer associate for the intellectual property firm Frommer, Lawrence & Haug in New York City, she learned about the patent and regulatory issues faced by companies, inventors, and researchers developing new pharmaceuticals and biotechnology. Now second vice president of NJPhA, she will become NJPhA president.

Personal Statement

I became interested in leadership and advocacy after learning about the unfortunate dichotomy between my clinical education and the practice of pharmacy in New Jersey. I felt the need to take action, get involved, and give the American community a broader recognition of the role of pharmacists. My family has been my support system throughout my pharmacy education. My father is a pharmacist and motivated me to enroll in pharmacy school; my mother is a nurse and has inspired me to use my talents to care for patients; and my sister is now in pharmacy school and has taught me the value of persistence and determination. Their constant encouragement has enabled me to pursue my goals in getting involved with leadership and advocacy.

My communication and coalition-building skills have served me best in my role as an advocate, but one mistake I have made and continue to make is doubting my idealistic goals. I became involved in leadership and advocacy because I thought one person could make a difference. At times, though, I am frustrated by practitioner apathy, ill-advised policy decisions, and the slow pace of change in practice. When I begin to doubt my idealism, I come one step closer to the apathy that can create a static profession. Pharmacy has been and must continue to be a dynamic profession.

Since my professional life does not end at 5 pm every day, I have had to learn to effectively manage my time. I regularly rely on my membership in professional associations, particularly NJPhA and APhA, for advocacy resources.

Most often, these invaluable experiences occur outside the classroom or library. A student does not learn how to be a pharmacist or a leader in the community by sitting at a desk or transcribing concepts onto countless index cards. Opportunities to apply their knowledge through interactions with mentors, patients, health care providers, and colleagues enhance students' learning experiences.

But balancing class work and outside experiences can be a challenge. Often, student leaders feel pressure from many sides. They must deal with personal obligations and financial concerns while trying to master professional-level course material, and making time for experience beyond the classroom may seem impossible. Thus, some students never pursue this valuable aspect of their education; they graduate without the practical skills to serve patients optimally and to advance the profession of pharmacy.

All student pharmacists, regardless of their future practice settings and lifestyles, are working toward the goal of graduating from a PharmD program. All of them have the potential to develop the skills to serve the public and the knowledge to ease human suffering. It is their exposure to practical experiences that makes the difference between simply adapting to the status quo and being crazy enough to change the world. The following stories of Andrew, Vibhuti, and Heather illustrate paths to becoming a future pharmacy leader. The experiences of these students provide valuable lessons about finding your passion, managing your time, and setting appropriate goals—essential elements for effective student leadership development.

Do More than Just Your Job

Andrew Traynor began pharmacy school in September 2000 at the University of Minnesota. Andy grew up on a dairy farm in Wisconsin, where he learned the value of taking pride in his work. "Do more than just your job. Strive for so much more than that," Andy's parents taught him. In high school, Andy searched for a fulfilling future career through a job-shadowing program. Having a family friend who was a pharmacist, Andy spent a day at a small rural hospital. There he noticed the pharmacist inter-acting with other health care professionals. Andy liked the idea of being a part of the health care team and applying medication knowledge, and he applied to pharmacy school.

During his first week of school, Andy remembers, faculty members and more experienced students emphasized the impor-tance of getting involved. He thought participating in school activities would help advance his career goals, as well as adding a philanthropic aspect to his new life as a college student. "My desire to give back came from my parents' idea of taking pride in what I do. To take pride in my schoolwork, I needed to give back as a way of reminding myself why I was at school." Partici-pating in student activities helped Andy to acclimate to college life, interact with colleagues, and establish his vision as a future pharmacist.

In his preprofessional years, Andy perceived that a community pharmacy was more a business than a place of patient care. On entering his first professional year of pharmacy school, however, his picture of a pharmacist shifted from that of a businessman to a health care provider. Andy learned that "a vision is something that is never set in stone and is always changing." Through his Introduction to Pharmaceutical Care class, Andy learned the con-cepts and philosophy of a patient-centered approach to practice. "Pharmacy was no longer limited to dealing with a commodity," he realized. "I learned there was something else out there."

Through his practice experience activities during school, Andy witnessed the impact his knowledge could have on someone's life. Visiting senior citizens' homes to talk about outdated medi-cations, explain medication risks, and answer questions, Andy began to appreciate the role of pharmacists. "For the first time, I realized that I had something to give, that how I spoke and listened to patients mattered." Combining this experience with his enhanced involvement in the American Pharmacists Asso-ciation–Academy of Student Pharmacists (APhA-ASP), Andy became inspired by the possibilities of his chosen profession. He realized the multifaceted role of a pharmacist.

In the spring of 2000, Andy attended his first APhA national meeting. Equipped with his classroom knowledge of pharmacy, he entered the student house of delegates session and was mes-merized by seeing students from across the country debating important issues for the profession. Attending this meeting was a life-altering event, Andy said. "At the house of delegates session, I kept thinking, 'If I don't do something, who will?'" With a sense of urgency, Andy approached his chapter advisor and professor, Todd Sorensen, during the meeting. He asked for advice on becoming actively involved. From that point, Andy took a greater leadership role in his APhA-ASP chapter.

> *It is a student's exposure to practical experiences that makes the difference between adapting to the status quo and being crazy enough to change the world.*

His story does not end here. The road to leadership presents challenges, especially to students in a rigorous PharmD program. "There is always that uneasy feeling in your stomach. How am I going to balance all this with my grades and social life? What am I getting myself into?" Luckily, Andy had faculty members and colleagues who supported his efforts. Andy's participation in extracurricular activities did not isolate him from his friends, since most of his friends were also involved in school professional organizations. Furthermore, his school administration and faculty encouraged involvement in outside experiences and accommodated academic schedules to allow students to attend workshops and meetings. "My dean and associate deans emphasized the importance of students communicating their needs so they could help us balance schoolwork with profession-building activities. I remember them saying, 'Let us know your schedule, if you need a tutor—whatever we can do to help, let us know.'"

The school's encouragement and the mentorship of a professor aided Andy in his success as a student leader. For example, Andy and his classmates' final exam in infectious diseases conflicted with attendance at the 2003 APhA annual meeting. Instead of discouraging their involvement in the meeting, the university allowed the students to take the exam when they returned. Andy says this action by the school reinforced the honor code, giving students the opportunity to engage in ethical practices while in school. The school trusted its students and treated them as future pharmacists, and Andy and his colleagues, in turn, learned the same respect toward the university and the profession.

A variety of events influenced Andy's development as a future pharmacist and leader in the community. "The best learning experiences are the ones that don't go so well," Andy said, noting that he developed his professional skill set through difficult decisions and occasional mistakes. For example, when he became president-elect of APhA-ASP, Andy initiated a change in the student awards process with the help of students on the awards committee. He envisioned an enhanced awards process that recognized more schools and students. In hindsight, however, he realized that the change was probably implemented too fast. "The big mistake was making the change without focusing on the interests of the different stakeholders, particularly the students themselves. Some students and advisors closely involved with the awards process did not like the change and were not given the opportunity to comment on the new process until after it was implemented."

Andy applied what he learned from that experience when he later worked with members of the student academy to change its name to be consistent with APhA's new name. Rather than having the matter decided at a national student executive meeting, Andy and the other national officers worked to communicate the idea to students throughout the country and solicit their opinions. After a 2-year discussion among students in their respective schools, the name change passed in the house of delegates. "I learned to improve upon my communication with stakeholders and to modify my vision on the basis of what I learned from them," Andy reflects.

These leadership lessons transferred to patient care situations during Andy's ambulatory care rotation. There, he met a patient who was confused about the price of his medications. Unable to pay for the medications, the patient was distraught. "I kept thinking, 'Realize his perspective, try to understand what he is going through; the patient is the stakeholder,'" said Andy. "That's when I thought of creating a system for discussing patient assistance programs." Andy was inspired to collaborate with practitioners at his rotation site on a system for better handling drug-related questions and problems for this ambulatory care population.

After pharmacy school, Andy completed the University of Minnesota's Pharmaceutical Care Leadership residency program. He continues to enhance his leadership skills and remembers the lessons he learned in pharmacy school, desiring to "pay his experiences forward."

Find a Passion but Also a Balance

Far from Andy's farm in Wisconsin, a 10-year-old girl named Vibhuti Arya moved to Washington Heights in New York City from New Delhi, India. Beginning a new life in America with her family, Vibhuti learned firsthand the struggles of being an immigrant. This experience continues to fuel her motivation to excel. "The journey has definitely been a challenge because I can't let my family's struggles be in vain," she said.

To this end, Vibhuti was determined to continue her education after high school. "Applying to pharmacy school was not my initial plan. I had little exposure to the profession and made the decision through high school recruitment." Vibhuti enrolled at St. John's University School of Pharmacy in the fall of 2000.

During her preprofessional years, Vibhuti became involved in several campus organizations. Remembering how much time she devoted to those activities, Vibhuti recalls an instance in which she could have used better communication. One evening while she was a residence assistant (RA), Vibhuti left a telephone message asking a staff member to cover her shift for an hour while she prepared for an exam. Unfortunately, the message was missed, the shift was not covered, and no responsible person was available during that hour, when the master locks for the building needed to be changed. Vibhuti realized she had not effectively balanced her RA and student roles. She should have spoken directly to the residence director in charge about her exam commitment. Vibhuti remembers this as a valuable lesson in time management, communication, and accountability. "It's hard to say no, especially when you want to put your all into your responsibilities, but you end up neglecting other priorities. I learned that you need to make time for yourself, your studies, and your other obligations." Vibhuti was a quick learner, and soon thereafter she was honored as RA of the month.

At the start of her first professional year at St. John's, Vibhuti's concept of the pharmacy profession was limited to the pharmacist's drug distribution role. Although shadowing programs in the previous years had exposed her to practice sites in hospitals, long-term care facilities, and community pharmacies, these visits focused on the delivery of medications rather than on patient care. Not until she met a student pharmacist named Bijal Sheth did Vibhuti begin learning pharmacists' broader role in health care. Through this student mentor, Vibhuti became involved in APhA-ASP. Meeting student pharmacists from other parts of the country and hearing their stories of pharmacists providing patient care made Vibhuti a believer. Joining the APhA-ASP Resolutions Committee, she worked to create policy goals related to the patient care aspect of pharmacy practice. "The Northeast is not the best place to witness patient care in pharmacies," Vibhuti admits. "While the concept exists, many practice sites have not embraced this role of pharmacists. Restrictive state laws that inhibit these activities here don't help, either."

Back at St. John's, Vibhuti shared her newfound knowledge with colleagues. "Most students in this area do not understand the concept of patient care in practice, because their exposure is limited," she said. "When I talk to students, they are surprised how pharmacy practice differs in other areas of the country, but they easily dismiss this reality because they are unable to witness it." Vibhuti believed this attitude was a barrier to greater involvement of students at her school. She feared these students would fail to develop the necessary skills to advance patient care.

Furthermore, she realized, "Being a pharmacist takes competence not only academically but also culturally. Some of my peers have yet to make a connection between school and the patient community." Vibhuti has a goal of educating students and health care professionals in the area of cultural competence. In New York, she has worked in pharmacies with diverse patient populations. Being an immigrant has helped her relate to patients who have difficulty understanding medication use because of language barriers or different customs. During her first rotation at a hospital clinic, Vibhuti discovered the extent of the problem. Most of the patients who came to the clinic did not speak English. She noticed the effect of language barriers on health disparities throughout several rotation sites.

Vibhuti remembers one patient who had come to the emergency room with chest pain. The patient acted uncomfortable and confused because she could not speak English. Realizing that the patient could better understand assessment questions in Spanish, Vibhuti translated the information for her. She discovered that the patient's sublingual nitroglycerin tablets were outdated and subpotent and that the patient did not understand the medication's indication or how to use it. As she explained the drug's purpose, Vibhuti

The dedication, innovation, and compassion of student pharmacists are needed to shape the future of the profession.

understood the importance of cultural competence in ensuring patient safety.

Some colleagues have questioned her involvement in professional activities, but Vibhuti has always been supported by her close family and a core group of friends. This has been especially important during hard times: "During the first semester of my second professional year, I went through a 'quarter-life crisis.' I had seven major leadership roles on campus and was attending more meetings than classes. I was completely burned out at the end of the semester. I felt like things were falling apart. Mentally drained, I felt like I didn't want to do everything anymore." Vibhuti spent her winter holiday break relaxing at home. After talking with her mother about the rough semester, Vibhuti realized she needed to make more time for herself. She remembered her experiences as an RA and understood that she needed to reapply the lessons she had learned. Embracing a vision for change in her university, Vibhuti had overextended herself.

After that difficult semester, Vibhuti reflected on her habits and found that one of the activities she enjoyed most, reading, was no longer a part of her life. When she was overcommitted, she lost her "own self." "If you don't appreciate the activities you are doing, then they are not worth it," she says. "I want to make sure I am advancing myself in all aspects, including mind, body, and soul. For example, I feel less of a person when I am not advancing my own spirituality through my living. I want to make sure I have my priorities straight. You can look at it from the perspective of realigning yourself with what makes you feel good as a person."

Vibhuti narrowed her activities to those that mattered most to her. She served as APhA-ASP national president during her final years in pharmacy school. Since graduation she has pursued a career path that allows her to engage in her passion for improving public health.

Manage Time, Set Goals, Study Communication

Further south, another woman made her way to pharmacy school after weighing several career options. Determined and self-motivated, Heather Ferguson graduated from high school and initially enrolled in the University of Florida intending to become a biochemical engineer. After a semester of study, she realized that her chosen major did not provide the interaction with people that she desired. Heather switched programs and became a firefighter and paramedic. She worked 24-hour shifts followed by 48 hours off. Eager to learn, she worked on a hospital surgical floor during her free time.

At the hospital, Heather befriended a pharmacy supervisor who asked her to work part-time in the pharmacy department. Her roommate was a student pharmacist, and Heather decided to try that field. Subsequently, she worked as a pharmacy technician and loved the experience. Heather had found the profession she wanted to pursue, and she enrolled at the University of Georgia College of Pharmacy.

Despite her exposure to the health care field as a paramedic and pharmacy technician, Heather did not appreciate a pharmacist's role in patient care until her second professional year of school. "Upon entering pharmacy school, I had only a superficial knowledge of what pharmacists were actually doing. I thought health-system pharmacists just entered inpatient orders and made sure patients were not allergic to medications, while community pharmacists just entered information, poured, and counted." Not until her pharmacy professor collaborated with local physicians to form a free community clinic did Heather witness pharmacists interacting with health care providers and counseling patients. At the clinic, the physicians let the student pharmacists perform the initial screening, take vital signs, and complete a drug history for each patient. "It was a wonderful experience that brought future classes into perspective," says Heather.

The road to leadership presents challenges, especially to students in a rigorous PharmD program. You need to make time for yourself, your studies, and your other obligations.

At school, Heather met an outgoing, determined student who served as her school's APhA-ASP president. Not only did he have a passion for pharmacy, he had "excitement and energy that spread throughout the chapter," Heather recalls. She became inspired by his example to get involved. She had a supportive environment for her efforts to make a difference, and Heather soon found herself saying yes to everything. "I joined as many organizations as I could and became involved in as many activities as I could." Since she had never been involved in extracurricular activities before pharmacy school, Heather had to learn how to manage her time.

"I used to make 'to do' lists but still never seemed to get everything finished," she said. Heather had to learn to prioritize and to say no. After attending leadership workshops, she recognized that her habit of completing the easy tasks on her list first and putting off the hardest, most complex tasks until last was not optimal. "I would get several things checked off, so I felt temporarily gratified, but then I would be frantically trying to complete the remaining tasks before deadline." Participating in such workshops taught Heather how to better prioritize and manage her work.

Heather also had to learn how to set goals as a student leader. She attempted to create a direction for her professional organizations by identifying issues of importance to members and incorporating them into organizational initiatives. This was not easy, however, because the needs of her peers varied from year to year. In the first professional year of pharmacy school, students were highly motivated but lacked focus. "We had big dreams and wanted to do everything, but had trouble focusing our energy," she remembered. Though many things were accomplished, more could have been done through better goal setting. By the second year, the dynamics of the leadership had changed such that members of the organization were more motivated than the officers. Since the officers had diverse personalities, communication was difficult. The officers had trouble conversing without creating conflict. Meanwhile, the members were eager to engage in projects. "That year we had to team build and work on communication. The dominant, outspoken officers learned how to listen while the quiet, soft-spoken ones learned how to get their point across."

Heather learned that although not everyone has good communication skills, communication can be improved by attending courses and workshops. "Students may find these seminars boring or even borderline silly while they are participating in them, but they will definitely be helpful in trying to communicate with patients and peers," Heather says. Such courses teach students how to adapt communication strategies to the capabilities of others and how to adjust to situations in which others are unable or unwilling to communicate effectively. To prepare for leadership as a pharmacist, Heather valued training in resolving conflict and understanding different styles of communication.

Heather remembers a valuable assignment given to her and another student during their first professional year. The project required visiting a patient in an assisted-living facility to talk about medication use. During the first visit, Heather recorded information about an elderly woman's 22 medications, including how she took the prescriptions and whether she experienced any adverse effects. Heather and her partner spent that evening devising a new medication treatment plan, which they presented to their pharmacy professor the next day. During their next visit with the patient, Heather and her partner explained the new plan. Eventually they presented it to her physician, which led to discontinuance of three medications and a new dosing schedule that gave the patient more energy throughout the day. The elderly patient was so grateful that she invited Heather and her colleague to visit with her neighbors and answer their questions. "I felt wonderful at the end of this project. Without even realizing it at the time, my partner and I demonstrated a variety of leadership skills while helping this patient. We had to communicate with the patient and her doctor. We also had to present our plan to our professor, along with our outcome goals. As a result, we empowered our patient to take charge of her therapy."

Heather carried this experience with her through her pharmacy training. Serving as a national APhA-ASP member-at-large and speaker of the house, Heather continued building her leadership skills. Since graduation, she has worked in a variety of settings. She worked in ambulatory care at a tribal American Indian pharmacy and a community hospital outpatient pharmacy. In addition, she worked at a hospital that is a level 1 trauma center serving Alaska, Montana, Oregon, Idaho, and Washington.

You Can Make a Difference

Most student pharmacists end their training by reciting the words of the Oath of a Pharmacist at graduation: "I will embrace and advocate change in the profession of pharmacy that improves patient care." Whether or not students think they can change the world, they will be changing it as they practice pharmacy.

Equipping student pharmacists with leadership skills is invaluable. Ours is not a profession that adopts a static attitude toward patient care. The dedication, innovation, and compassion of student pharmacists are needed to shape the future of the profession. The three student leaders discussed here have moved on to productive professional careers. As they continue to build their leadership skills, they remember the lessons they learned in pharmacy school. The following story, derived from Loren Eiseley's *The Star Thrower*, captures the lessons that Andrew, Vibhuti, and Heather teach:

> A man walking along a beach noticed a child throwing starfish into the ocean. The man asked, "Why are you throwing starfish in the ocean?" The child answered, "The sun is rising and the tide is going out. If I don't throw them in, they'll die." The man replied, "But don't you know there are miles and miles of beach with starfish all along it? You can't possibly make a difference." The young boy listened politely, then picked up another starfish and threw it into the ocean, stating, "It made a difference for that one."

LEADERSHIP MENTORING

Mary L. Euler

The need for leadership development in pharmacy has been well documented. As pharmacists' roles continue to evolve and practice opportunities expand, our profession must be vigilant in charting the course for our future. The vision of change that has carried us through the past three decades must continue if we wish to assume a role in patient care that will lead to a healthier society. We must ensure that our future leaders are prepared to face the challenges of internal and external forces working to undermine the education and training that have brought us to this exciting time in our profession's history.

The responsibility for leadership training should be felt in practice, academia, and associations; each has a role to play in identifying, training, and mentoring our next generation of leaders. Every current leader should have as a goal the training of his or her replacement, in preparation for moving into a new role or retirement. Leadership should not happen by accident but through well-planned educational and training programs, facilitated and supported by effective mentoring relationships.

Mary L. Euler

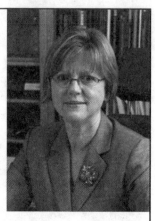

Background

Mary Euler has served as Executive Director of Phi Lambda Sigma (PLS), the pharmacy leadership society, since 2000. In this capacity she provides the administrative foundation for the PLS Executive Board and 81 chapters in the United States and Puerto Rico. She is Assistant Dean of the University of Missouri–Kansas City (UMKC) School of Pharmacy, overseeing alumni affairs, development, and the professional degree satellite program in Columbia. For 13 years she served as UMKC's American Pharmacists Association–Academy of Student Pharmacists (APhA-ASP) advisor and in 1997 received the APhA-ASP Outstanding Chapter Advisor Award. For her work in student mentoring, Euler was also honored with the 2003 Gloria Niemeyer Francke Leadership Mentor Award. She has received the Missouri Pharmacy Association's Pharmacist Making a Difference Award, UMKC's Matthew W. "Bill" Wilson Alumnus of the Year Award, and several community service awards for her work to improve the lives of the underserved in Kansas City.

Personal Statement

My parents taught me that I was responsible for the choices I made in life. When I chose pharmacy as a career, that lesson naturally followed into my professional life, and I entered my career knowing that I was ultimately responsible for my profession.

Leadership and advocacy require understanding the issue or problem at hand. To this end, there are no substitutes for active listening and research—and here is where my mistakes have occurred. In my early, more ambitious years, I tended to act too quickly and sometimes missed the target. The greatest lesson I have learned from advocacy and leadership development is respect for the value of others. I delegate easily because I trust that others can do a job as well as or better than I can, and this has made my personal and professional life much more manageable.

The Role of the Mentor

The role of mentoring in leadership development overshadows all other formal and informal training programs. It is not enough for schools and colleges of pharmacy to simply teach courses in practice management theory or for associations to offer leadership development programs. The concept of "use it or lose it" applies when students and new practitioners are not given the opportunities and support necessary to try their newly learned skills on for size. To take the next step, many need the encouragement and safety net provided by a mentor. Without mentoring relationships, many aspiring leaders will be left behind at a time when pharmacy can ill afford to overlook their potential for advancing our profession.

Much has been written about the role of the mentor in learning relationships. *The Mentor's Guide* by Lois Zachary[1] offers a context for the relationship between learners and mentors, a structure that can help mentors understand how their role as facilitators allows learners or mentees to take the active role in the process of reaching their goals. Zachary's guide is one of many tools available for current and would-be mentors. It is important for those who mentor to have a basic understanding of their place in the relationship. I expect, however, that most pharmacy mentors, like me, have not had the luxury of formal study. Rather, they step into the role out of a desire to help others achieve their goals and thus ensure advancement of the profession.

My own journey into mentorship was more accidental than planned. Shortly after my start as a new faculty member, our American Pharmacists Association–Academy of Student Pharmacists (APhA-ASP) president approached me in the hallway and asked if I would be the new chapter advisor. Eager to please and a little naive, I quickly said yes and thus began my mentoring journey, and a great one it has been. Although I did not set out to become a mentor, I did take an oath upon graduation to work to advance my profession. Being a mentor has allowed me a far greater reach than I could have had on my own. In essence, mentoring expands the capacity for leadership in our profession. By instilling in student pharmacists a sense of responsibility and a desire to lead, mentors provide for the future of our profession, encouraging others to develop their skills, seek opportunities, and accept leadership positions.

The Need for Leadership Development

The past 30 years have been a time of much change in our profession—some good and some not so good. By facilitating the leadership development of pharmacy students, we can feel confident that pharmacy will continue to be a driving force in the health care system. A 2005 survey of pharmacy managers, practitioners, and pharmacy students published in the *American Journal of Health-System Pharmacy*[2] revealed the following:

- In the next decade, we will need 4,000 to 5,000 new directors of pharmacy and other managers to account for the retirement of current leaders in those areas.
- Only 44% of those retiring managers would recommend a current staff member to replace their position.
- Even if offered such a position, it is unclear whether many pharmacists would accept it; only 30% of current practitioners in the areas surveyed indicated an interest in seeking leadership positions. This news seems dire.
- The survey revealed that 62% of pharmacy students aspired to leadership positions, and that number provides great hope for the future.

Using only a conservative estimate of approximately 10,000 students currently enrolled, we have 6,200 students interested in leadership positions. We cannot abandon the 30% in current positions who have the talent, motivation, and experience needed for leadership, but we must give considerable attention to the 62% in our schools and colleges of pharmacy who aspire to leadership.

It is unrealistic for us to believe that student pharmacists and young practitioners will become the leaders of tomorrow simply through desire or through having held elected office in school or attended leadership development programs. The road to leadership requires opportunities to use what has been learned through meaningful and well-planned itineraries under the guidance of mentors. Opportunities for such training are available, but often they are difficult for the aspiring leader to find or access. Mentors, through their own networks, can help bridge this gap. If aspiring leaders cannot find opportunities and they believe opportunities do not exist or think their talents are not needed, they quickly lose the interest, enthusiasm, and confidence they once had for leadership. This is a great loss to our profession. Sadly, this phenomenon occurs many times every year as once-active student leaders graduate from pharmacy school. The structure and support for continued growth are gone. Rather than being recruited for their leadership skills, these graduates are recruited as employees and members.

Strategies for Developing Mentoring

Pharmacy associations that keep track of their former student leaders and encourage their participation on committees, task forces, and new practitioner initiatives are to be commended for their efforts to create and mentor a pipeline of leaders, but so much more can be done. Local and state associations should be waiting in the wings to recruit and mentor their future leaders upon graduation. Pharmacy employers should maintain close contact with schools and colleges of pharmacy, as well as residency programs, to recruit not only for vacant positions but for leadership potential. Academia should put much greater effort into preparing faculty for leadership positions and should recognize leadership development as having substantial importance in promotion and tenure processes. As new practitioners with leadership interest enter the workforce, they should be met by mentors who will guide them to the next level. Leadership development in the workplace should be a component of every employment contract and should not be viewed as something pharmacists do on the side for their own benefit.

At every level, pharmacists should not be forced to use personal time to provide service to their profession or participate in programs that aid the advancement of the profession. We cannot continue to criticize our current and new practitioners for not seeking leadership positions if they have not been provided the support and training necessary to be successful. Whether or not we remember this, someone helped us reach our goals, and now it's payback time—although I prefer to see it as fulfilling our responsibility to pharmacy.

Perhaps this is not a traditional mentoring role, but those interested in promoting leadership development in pharmacy should work diligently to identify leadership potential among our students and young practitioners. Leaders can be found in unlikely places. Leaders are not just those extroverted individuals who self-identify, but also those who sit quietly listening to the needs of others. They may have the passion but lack the confidence to participate. A good mentor can help those less confident individuals find a purpose and become contributors to pharmacy leadership. In my experience, those in the latter group require more encouragement but can, with support and validation, use their skills to become effective leaders. We cannot afford to leave them behind.

When considering leadership potential, we need to look for skills in others that would help round out an effective leadership team. Such skills include active listening, analysis and problem solving, organizational and time management, and delegation, as well as execution of

> *The responsibility for leadership training should be felt in practice, academia, and associations; each has a role to play in identifying, training, and mentoring our next generation of leaders.*

activities and tasks. Rarely can all of these skills be found in one individual; rather, each person has a few prominent traits and can benefit from the strengths of others. Mentors can help mentees identify their own strengths while accepting that others may have needed qualities that they lack. Creating an effective leadership team goes a long way toward preventing team members from feeling overburdened—a feeling that causes individuals to not seek leadership roles or ultimately to leave them. It does not have to be lonely at the top. Behind every good leader is an equally good but different style of leader. Mentors can help mentees find a leadership style that fits their own strengths.

Aspiring leaders seek mentors for a variety of reasons. For example, many are looking for mentors to help them sort out their strengths, areas for improvement, and goals in supportive environments. Mentors can provide a nonjudgmental environment that allows open and candid discussion, self-assessment, and encouragement. At no time can the mentor's role be more critical than at times when a leadership pursuit fails. The energy and enthusiasm of those who are unsuccessful in their attempt to assume leadership positions can easily be lost forever without the support of a mentor who can help them analyze, refocus, and set new leadership goals. For example, a student who loses an election might feel rejected, discouraged, and disappointed. Mentors can provide assurance that the leadership development process is a longitudinal experience—a series of events from which we learn and grow.

Challenges in Finding a Mentor

During the past 19 years I have had the opportunity to work with aspiring student leaders across the country through my involvement in APhA-ASP and Phi Lambda Sigma, the pharmacy leadership society. Early on, these relationships were most often local, but advances in technology have allowed relationships with students far from my home in the Midwest. With a strong preference for the personal touch, I never thought I would allow myself to become a "virtual" mentor, but I have found that students and young practitioners are eagerly seeking individuals, regardless of location, for encouragement and support as they try to hone their leadership skills. No longer does the mentor have to be a close personal contact, faculty member, or employer. Although long-distance mentoring relationships have an element of risk, they have great value for the mentee who cannot find an appropriate mentor close to home. Current mentors can facilitate these virtual relationships through their network of colleagues.

Furthermore, mentors should always recognize their own limitations and know when to refer a mentee to someone who is better suited to help. This can be hard, especially for mentors who have invested a great deal of time and personal commitment. Letting go is a necessary and selfless act that provides closure or growth in other directions. I enjoy hearing from former mentees who have found what they were seeking and also remember me for the part I may have played in their professional success. For many of us in pharmacy, this is all the reward we need for mentoring.

Conclusion

In his book *Even Eagles Need a Push*, David McNally states that "what distinguishes truly successful people is that they are contributors....their accomplishments, their successes, are rooted in their desire to be of service to humanity."[3] Those who have accepted the responsibility of mentoring have a desire to serve. Mentors are contributors who find their success through the success of others and in doing so serve the greater good. Mentors are role models and leaders who are not threatened by the success of others and, in fact, work to train their replacements.

All too often, when people think of leaders they think only of those who have been elected to office. However, leadership takes many forms in our profession. The many leadership roles can provide diverse experiences for developing leaders, and the demand for leadership will grow as the profession expands. Pharmacy managers in hospitals, community practice, academia, long-term care, mail order, managed care, and all settings have the same important responsibility for leadership in the profession as those who serve in high-level positions through elected or appointed office in our associations. But many pharmacists and student pharmacists are ill prepared to assume these leadership roles; the road to these positions is more often serendipitous than systematic. Thus, pharmacy needs more mentors to help identify, encourage, support, and open doors for our future leaders. I cannot imagine any greater contribution we can make to pharmacy.

References

1. Zachary L. *The Mentor's Guide: Facilitating Effective Learning Relationships.* San Francisco: Jossey-Bass; 2000.
2. White SJ. Will there be a pharmacy leadership crisis? *Am J Health Syst Pharm.* 2005;62:845–55.
3. McNally D. *Even Eagles Need a Push.* New York: Dell Publishing; 1990.

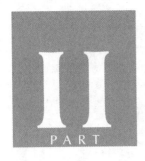

PART

APPLYING ADVOCACY FOR PHARMACY

Making the Transition from Leadership to Advocacy

John M. O'Brien

I n previous chapters of this book, current pharmacy leaders who have known, studied, and learned from pharmacy's greatest leaders offer their experiences and suggestions for developing as an effective leader and encouraging pharmacists to get involved. One of a leader's greatest skills is the ability to encourage others to believe they are capable of accomplishing their goals. An effective leader will help you see pharmacy's rich history and how far we've advanced. He or she will also help you see that pharmacists are the answer to some of the health care system's greatest unmet needs.

The leaders from whom I've been lucky enough to learn—both in person and in print—have made me feel like a football player waiting to take the field before the Super Bowl. Think about the last time you saw that scene—a group of athletes, all dressed the same, bouncing up and down with excitement in their eyes— all ready to work together to win the game. If leadership is the speech in the locker room, then advocacy is what happens after kickoff.

John Michael O'Brien

Background

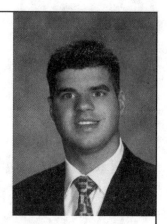

John O'Brien is President of Responsible Health, LLC, a public health consulting practice that works with patient groups, provider organizations, policy makers, and prescription drug manufacturers to design public health initiatives that teach health literacy, increase access to medicine, improve health outcomes, and lower health care costs. He is a former Senior Director of State Policy at the Pharmaceutical Research and Manufacturers of America (PhRMA) and worked with state officials to improve the affordability of medications and access to prescription drugs. He is a health care futurist and lectures frequently about Medicare, Medicaid, evidence-based medicine, consumer-driven health care, and the uninsured. Before joining PhRMA, he worked in the Medical and Scientific Affairs and Government Affairs departments of Sankyo Pharma Inc., now Daiichi Sankyo.

O'Brien was the 2000–2001 Executive Resident in Association Management and Leadership at the American Society of Health-System Pharmacists (ASHP). He completed the Master of Public Health degree and Certificate in Health Policy and Management program at the Johns Hopkins Bloomberg School of Public Health, where he currently serves as a faculty associate. He earned a Doctor of Pharmacy degree from Nova Southeastern University after studying pharmacy and political science at the University of Florida. As a student, he was an American Medical Student Association Washington Health Policy Fellow, an American Society of Consultant Pharmacists Paul Cano Legislative Intern, and an American Pharmacists Association–Academy of Student Pharmacists (APhA-ASP) regional delegate.

Personal Statement

I became interested in leadership and advocacy when a pharmacist mentor told me that if I was unhappy with what I saw, then I either had to get involved or get used to it. I was lucky to have Charlie Bucalo, Theresa Wells Tolle, Kathy Petsos, Norm Tomaka, and Mark Hobbs as early mentors, all in the same county pharmacy association. Since then, I've been blessed to have learned from some of pharmacy's and health care's most influential leaders and advocates.

The most effective technique I've learned is the value of storytelling. Though my friends and my wife are certainly sick of hearing them, I tell stories to make my points. Stories engage people, and they are more valuable than lecturing or preaching in the first person.

The biggest mistake I've made is wanting things to happen too quickly. I have Dr. Joe Oddis to thank for this lesson. From him I learned when an idea should stay in the briefcase and when it should be pulled out.

Henri Manasse, Lucinda Maine, and Billy Tauzin have all taught me that being a servant first and a leader second transcends everything else. I strive to be a trusted collaborator who listens to and supports others, more than a leader interested only in power, prestige, and the material trappings of leadership.

I passionately believe the stars are lining up for pharmacists to improve the health care system, and I thank the countless leaders and members of the pharmacy profession who have had the patience and tolerance to mentor me and listen to me.

The transition from leadership to advocacy is simply communicating what you believe and helping other stakeholders believe it too. The contributors in this section of the book define effective advocacy and describe how it can be applied for positive results. By practicing effective advocacy, individual pharmacists and pharmacy organizations will be able to achieve the goals that pharmacy leaders have helped them to see.

Advocacy in Pharmacy and Health Care

"Since you spend more time with your patients than their physician does, why don't you get paid for it?" the Florida-based pharmacy intern inquired.

"Do you know the Golden Rule?" Dr. Bucalo asked. "Whoever has the gold makes the rules."

"That's not right," said the intern. "Someone should do something about it."

"Knock yourself out," Dr. Bucalo replied. "The people to talk to are in Tallahassee."

The history of health care is full of political milestones affecting health professionals and the patients they serve. The Flexner Report of 1910 changed the face of medical education and the future of osteopathic medicine. The Medicare and Medicaid programs created health care for the aged, disabled, and poor in 1964. Congress granted nurse practitioners and registered dietitians Medicare provider status in 1997 and 2000. These events did not just occur; they were influenced by individual and collective advocacy on behalf of and in opposition to the causes of many different stakeholders.

Advocacy is the active support of an idea, cause, or position. Health care advocates may seek to expand services to patients, protect the interests of businesses, expand a scope of practice for providers, or change the way a group or cause is viewed by others. Advocates may be professionals paid to support a cause or volunteers representing their own cause. The chapters that follow discuss advocacy in its many forms, styles, and arenas. However, effective advocacy in all instances involves delivering your message to opinion leaders, elected officials, decision makers, or those who can help you influence them. Whether you communicate during a personal visit, through an article in a major newspaper, or at a rally on the steps of the statehouse, if your message isn't concise, credible, convincing, and heard by someone in a position to influence the outcome you seek, it won't make a difference.

The message you deliver may be the most important part of advocacy development. Effective message development requires knowing the facts, making them your own, and telling a story that interests the people you're trying to influence. In marketing, emotions are at the top of the ladder of benefits. BMW doesn't sell cars by talking about the specifications of its engines or the functional performance of its cars; it sells "the ultimate driving machine."[1] Volvo appeals to a different buyer by "building cars with you in mind" and conveying a feeling of safety for you and your family. Air bags are necessary features, and crash test ratings measure functional performance, but "fitting your family's needs securely" sells emotion to people who value keeping their family safe and comfortable. Both BMW and Volvo convey a feeling to different consumers with different values. Because each stakeholder or decision maker is different, the same message often has to be delivered in slightly different ways. This applies to pharmacy as well. Patients expect the facts when they receive patient advisory leaflets with their prescriptions. They expect functional performance—for their medications to work. But most important, they trust pharmacists, who are responsible for optimizing outcomes to keep them safe.

The Role of Storytelling in Advocacy

Emotions are also at the top of the ladder of advocacy. During your legislative visit, a Senate staffer may listen to you and may write down your comments: "Pharmacists are drug therapy experts; they go to school for 6 to 8 years; preventable medication errors are the fifth leading cause of death and cost between $85 billion and $177 billion per year." Whether your talking points ever leave the staffer's notes is another story.

Imagine that during your introduction you talked with that staffer for a moment about your mutual hometown. Perhaps when you asked about family, the staffer told you about his child who likes soccer, or about her best friend who recently had a stroke. Also imagine that instead of repeating your talking points, you told a story about the time you caught a potential drug–drug interaction before it happened to an elderly person back home, shared how the asthma counseling you provide every day helped a 10-year-old girl play soccer again, or discussed how the anticoagulation services you provide mean the difference between stroke-causing blood clots or a robust quality of life. Which approach do you think will be more likely to get the staffer to advocate for your cause with his or her legislator?

Mutually Shared Benefits, or Getting What You Want by Giving Others What They Want

In a perfect world, the health care system would recognize pharmacists' abilities to improve patient outcomes and decrease total health care costs, and pharmacists would be paid for their services. Instead, pharmacy's advocacy campaign has focused on informing decision makers that pharmacists are trained medication experts who work collaboratively with patients and physicians to improve medication use. Progress, albeit slow, is being made toward payment for pharmacists' services, with government programs such as Medicare and with private payers. The gains realized are due to the efforts of many, and those gains must be monitored and amplified. The mutually shared benefits are reduced costs for health care and payment for pharmacists' patient care services separate from order fulfillment.

The Role of Shared Goals

Another strategy is to help others see how pharmacists can help them achieve their goals. A favorite story involves a petroleum engineer who wanted to break into the oil shipping business.[2] Rafael Tudela, at the time a Venezuelan glass manufacturer, learned that the Argentinean government was investigating a $20 million purchase of butane. Tudela bid against experienced energy companies British Petroleum and Shell Oil for the contract. He was also aware that Argentina was desperately trying to sell an oversupply of beef. So he offered to sell Argentina the butane and buy $20 million worth of its beef. He was awarded the contract only if he could take delivery of the beef at closing. Tudela also knew that Spain was facing political pressure related to the closing of a shipyard, and he offered to build a $20 million supertanker at the shipyard if Spain would buy $20 million worth of beef. Spain readily agreed and immediately arranged for Argentina to ship Tudela's beef directly across the Atlantic. Tudela then traveled to Sun Oil's Philadelphia headquarters and offered to buy $20 million of butane if they would charter his soon-to-be-completed supertanker. Tudela, armed only with the knowledge of what other people wanted, was able to outmaneuver more experienced and established competitors, fulfilling his dream of entering the oil business, and building a billion-dollar business in less than 20 years.

It may be impossible to find a stakeholder that wants only to see pharmacists reimbursed for their services. In fact, other health care stakeholders may be working against pharmacy because they fear losing control of the prescribing process or losing the revenue they earn in the current system. What would happen if pharmacists identified allies who also wanted to reduce health care spending, improve quality, and ensure appropriate use of prescription drugs? Pharmacists could help them achieve shared goals.

The Role of Collaboration

When I feel the heat, I see the light.

—Former Senate Majority Leader Everett Dirksen

A variation on getting what you want by giving someone else what he or she wants involves convincing other stakeholders that you support the same theme, if not the same issue. Some of the most successful lobbying and advocacy campaigns in history have been conducted by building issue campaigns with other organizations. Having other organizations deliver *your* message as *their* message is very powerful, especially if the other organization is more politically numerous or coveted.

> *Whether you are behind the counter or in front of the Senate, if you are willing and able to convince others to believe what you believe, you have made the transition from leadership to advocacy.*

The Medicare Catastrophic Coverage Act (MCCA) of 1988 offered increased benefits to Medicare beneficiaries, including coverage of outpatient prescription drugs. A key provision of the legislation required Medicare beneficiaries with higher incomes to pay a supplemental premium tax. Although only 5% of seniors would pay the maximum tax, opponents of MCCA were able to enrage seniors about this provision and enlist their help in working toward its repeal. AARP, which enjoyed early accolades for working with Congress to improve benefits for seniors, began receiving 50,000 letters of opposition for every 30 letters of support.

One spectacular event involving a public display of outrage by seniors helped lead to the 1989 repeal of MCCA. The situation involved Representative Dan Rostenkowski (D-IL), the chair of the House Ways and Means Committee and an author of the bill, who was returning to his home district to discuss senior advocates' concerns at a senior center. During the meeting private negotiations broke down, and Rep. Rostenkowki exited the building to find sign-waving seniors calling him a liar and a chicken. When he and his staff began to drive away, an elderly woman wearing rose-colored, heart-shaped glasses jumped onto the hood of his car until her face was pressed against the windshield. Rostenkowski ran from the car and cut through a gas station to get away, while the cameras rolled and captured the angry protestors' chants of "Coward!" and "Impeach him!"

Some may question the role of special interests in organizing the seniors and the tactics they used to garner support for the repeal of MCCA. However, no one disputes the impact of national news images of a 15-term representative running from angry seniors. The next time lawmakers propose policies that undermine pharmacists' ability to help patients, who will be angry enough to protest on your behalf?

Advocacy Happens Anywhere, Anytime, and One Person at a Time

Consider the following actual situation:

"So, whatta you do?" said the gentleman in the seat next to the pharmacist during a transcontinental flight.

"I'm a clinical pharmacist," the pharmacist replied. "I help people make better use of their medicine."

"How do you do that? Do you have a specialty?"

That simple icebreaker turned into an extended conversation about what pharmacists do. During the conversation the pharmacist didn't cite facts or figures; he told stories. He talked about all the pharmacists he knew who are helping children avoid asthma attacks, seniors save money and live longer, happier lives, and business owners reduce health care costs. He used names and talked about communities. Shortly before the plane landed, the seatmate asked him a clinical question, the answer to which he e-mailed to his seatmate before they reached their final destination. Truth be told, that scenario has repeated itself many times, leading to relationships between pharmacists and legislators, social entrepreneurs, business owners, venture capitalists, and professional athletes. Once you have an individual's attention and are seen to be helpful to the person's cause, such random encounters can turn into meaningful relationships.

Walking Your Talk

Who you are speaks so loudly I can't hear what you're saying.

—Ralph Waldo Emerson

What would happen if your goal in every personal conversation about health care was to use emotions to advocate for pharmacists and better use of prescription medicines? Each pharmacist in each practice setting has opportunities to use emotions to advocate for the profession. You have countless examples of how you've helped patients. Have you ever thought about how you made your patients feel? Safe? Comforted?

Market research shows that when consumers are stressed, they seek products and services that make them feel safe and well. For example, in 2003, there was a 50% increase in sales of products that contain vanilla after several articles appeared in the lay literature that promoted its value.[3] Whether tasted or smelled, vanilla appears to create a feeling of comfort that soothes people. If confusion and anger are red and loud, then vanilla is white and quiet. With patients more frustrated and confused about drug costs, drug safety, and drug coverage choices, pharmacists have an opportunity to soothe them and make them feel safe and well. If your actions make people feel that they have nothing to be concerned about, and that they can leave the pharmacy feeling safe and well, they will seek your services (and recommend them to others). If their fears make them "go red," how can you soothe them?

Individual pharmacists also represent the profession as a whole. Imagine a legislator visiting a busy pharmacy on the first business day of 2006 and observing the following. Regular patients are returning from winter vacation and need refills of their medications; new patients are attempting to use their Medicare prescription drug coverage for the first time; and a caregiver comes in to ask questions about her parents' drug coverage. They are all upset about the new Part D program and are very confused. No one recognizes the Senator; she is simply standing at the counter with everybody else. However, she is observing how you handle these patient concerns. Would she see you blaming the circumstances on "those bureaucrats in Washington" and making the patients more red, or would she see you make them feel safe and well? Would she see the type of pharmacist who was sitting on the airplane in the previous example advocating for pharmacy?

Conclusion

If we fail to dare, if we do not try, the next generation will harvest the fruit of our indifference; a world we did not want—a world we did not choose—but a world we could have made better, by caring more for the results of our labors.

—Senator Robert F. Kennedy

The history of health care has been shaped by visionaries who saw how pharmacists could solve existing or future problems. These leaders long believed that pharmacy had the potential for an expanded scope of practice, and pharmacists today are helping patients in ways their predecessors could only dream about. The literature documents pharmacists improving patients' quality of care and decreasing health care costs, and policy makers and decision makers are looking to us for help. The stars are indeed lining up for pharmacists.

As you follow the leaders you believe in and as you lead and mentor others, you will have an opportunity to advocate for pharmacists and the patients they serve. You will have an opportunity to learn the strategies and tactics for lobbying and advocacy, and use them to show everyone you meet what you believe about pharmacists and their distinctive role in health care. Likewise, they will have an opportunity to advocate on your behalf. Whether you are behind the counter or in front of the Senate, if you are willing and able to convince others to believe what you believe, you have made the transition from leadership to advocacy.

This chapter has provided an overview of how advocacy stems from leadership. In the remaining chapters, specific information and examples will give you additional insight into this important process.

Are you a pharmacist, or are you a mouse?

—Professor Paul Doering

References

1. Silverstein M, Fiske N, Butman J. *Trading Up: Why Consumers Want New Luxury Goods*. New York: Portfolio; 2003.
2. McCormack M. *What They Don't Teach You at Harvard Business School: Notes from a Street-Smart Executive*. New York: Bantam; 1984:54–5.
3. Howard T. Vanilla: wear it, eat it, drink it, love it. *USA Today*. April 28, 2003.

MAKING AN IMPACT ON FEDERAL LEGISLATION

William G. Lang

I n *The Music Man*, Professor Harold Hill and his salesmen cronies keep repeating that "You've got to know the territory" before you can succeed. The same is true if you want to be an effective advocate. You have to know the legislative territory: who makes the decisions that affect pharmacy and health care, how the system works, and how you can make an impact. This chapter describes the legislative process and provides some strategies for working effectively within this complex process. Although you may be familiar with parts of the process, some of these ideas may be new to you.

Understanding How Congress Works

The U.S. Congress consists of two chambers, the Senate and the House of Representatives. Members of the two chambers are housed in buildings on the north and south sides of Capitol Hill, flanking the imposing Capitol building. The 100 Senators have offices in the Russell, Dirksen, and Hart office buildings, and the 435 members of the House, in the Rayburn, Longworth, and

William G. "Will" Lang

Personal Statement

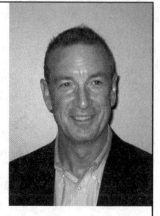

As the offspring of parents who were active in their community, I came to appreciate volunteerism at an early age. My initial activism revolved around county political party activities—which I always saw as a way to attend the county fair free of charge. I now know that once you are a volunteer, you will most likely remain a volunteer. Being an active participant in your community and advocating for your beliefs is extremely important and is a recognized part of being an American citizen. Taking the cue from my parents, their friends, and local leaders, I was able to develop relationships that provided opportunities for mentoring, increased exposure, and the nurturing of a lifelong interest in my surroundings.

Making a difference means developing and maintaining relationships with a wide network of individuals. Advocacy and leadership require the support of constituencies that share similar goals and beliefs. Meeting people who share your advocacy goals and maintaining those relationships is the most expedient way to build support for personal and group goals and agendas. As in any relationship, the need for truthful and forthright communication is essential. Building support for an advocacy agenda requires focused dedication to bringing to potential supporters' attention information and insight they may not get without your assistance.

Luckily for me, I learned, early in my career as an advocate, the importance of checking facts and figures myself before sharing them with potential supporters. There is nothing more personally distressing than to be challenged on the correctness of information you are presenting before a legislative committee. Once burned, I have always concerned myself with the authenticity and veracity of my information.

Early in the 18th century, the American way of community development and interaction was identified as unique. No other place has ever fostered the type of opportunities we have created for discussing shared issues and their resolution. My personal life has been greatly enhanced by the relationships I have initiated and maintained through community activities I have volunteered or advocated for. There is no greater satisfaction than knowing that your actions make a positive difference in the lives of others. Being an active member of society, no matter what the issue or cause, is more American than apple pie, and more lastingly satisfying.

Cannon office buildings. In these buildings are the members' personal offices, as well as committee rooms and offices for committee staff.

Unlike many state legislators, members of Congress have numerous staff members who assist them with a wide range of activities. Constituent services and public relations are important responsibilities of congressional staff, but even more important are ensuring that the member is aware of key issues and preparing the member for committee and floor work. The activity of each member's personal office is coordinated and managed by a chief of staff. Legislative initiatives introduced by or important to a member are supervised by the legislative director. Specific areas are handled by legislative assistants, who are responsible for meeting with constituents and representatives of special interest groups concerned with issues in the staff person's particular area (e.g., health, education, tax policy, defense, banking).

Every member of Congress sits on at least one committee. Committee appointments usually reflect a member's interest or expertise in the issues over which that committee has jurisdiction. Committee activity is overseen by the committee staff; both the majority and the minority party have staff support. As legislation is introduced, it is forwarded to the committee having jurisdiction in that subject area. To a great extent, the committee chair determines whether the introduced legislation will be brought before the committee for consideration. Legislation that languishes in committee can be petitioned for release, but this process is rarely initiated.

Committees hold hearings on specific issues that often lead to the development of legislation by the committee itself. Legislation developed through the committee process usually finds quicker acceptance and consideration by an individual chamber than does standalone legislation introduced by an individual member, regardless of the number of co-sponsors the legislation may have.

Once the hearings are held and legislation is created, the committee moves toward the "chair's mark." This is a formal presentation of the committee's work, with the opportunity for members to bring amendments for consideration by the chair. If a bill is successfully "marked up," it is then placed on the calendar of the respective chamber, and there it awaits the call of that chamber's leader, either the Speaker of the House or the Senate Majority Leader. When the respective leader deems it appropriate, the legislation is brought to the floor of the chamber, where members vote the legislation "up" or "down." Legislation passed in one chamber must then successfully complete this same process in the other chamber. If it is passed by both chambers, it goes to the President of the United States to be signed. Should the President "veto" the bill (refuse to sign it), Congress can still pass the legislation if two-thirds of each chamber votes to pass it.

Thousands of bills are introduced annually in any session of Congress. Only a small percentage of introduced legislation is ever passed into law; this is an affirmation of the important aspects of legislative rules and procedures and the deliberative nature of the process.

Prioritizing Your Time and Effort

Since the chance that a given bill will be passed is slim and the size of the enterprise is larger than ever before, how can citizens believe they can make an impact through advocacy? For an individual, the process seems unwieldy, fraught with undisclosed actions, and arcane in almost every aspect. At first, it seems nearly impossible to develop any skill in influencing legislation across such a vast organization with so many moving parts. This may be the case, but the good news is that advocacy is relatively easy if you start by learning the process and then prioritize your time and effort. Unless you are part of a very large organization, you must focus your attention on members of Congress, their staff, and the committees that act in your area of concern.

The best place to begin is with the member of the House who represents the congressional district in which you live and the two members of the Senate who represent your state. These are the members who should have the greatest interest in your issue or concern. Providing effective constituent services is the best way for a member of Congress to ensure re-election. These congressional offices are where you can gain valuable support and information as you continue your advocacy, and the most important step is developing and maintaining a relationship with the key staff in these offices. Regular contact with the staff dedicated to health care issues can give you valuable insight into congressional activity and priorities.

Always remember that as soon as you finish your conversation and walk out the office door or hang up the phone, the staffer will meet with or take a call from another constituent. You must continually keep your issue in front of the staffers. Keep them interested in your issues by sending them articles or editorials that reflect your position. Improve their awareness of your issue area by inviting them to see firsthand the impact of the issue back in your district. There is nothing more powerful than seeing a demonstration of or the impact of a process or program. For example, a visit to campus by an elected official or that person's staff members is the best way to help them understand and appreciate the intricacies of current pharmacy education.

As may be apparent, not all members of Congress are created equal. Whether the member is part of the majority or the minority party or sits on a committee with jurisdiction over your issue can make a huge difference in your efforts. Consideration of the member's seniority within committees is a good starting point. Of greatest influence are those members of Congress who chair committees. A chair is selected by the majority party leadership during the start of a congressional session. Chairs of committees that appropriate funding to federal agencies and programs are so highly respected that they are commonly referred to as "Cardinals." The chair of a committee calls the shots for consideration or nonconsideration of all the introduced legislation that has been deemed germane to the committee's jurisdictional areas.

The committee chair is supported by a large staff. The committee has a chief of staff who works closely with the chair and oversees committee staff. These staff members are traditionally divided into the jurisdictional issue areas of the committee. Like your own congressional delegation's office staff, the committee staff member who works on your issue is an important contact and potential ally. This individual may or may not have a significant understanding of and background on issues before the committee and rarely has the level of understanding that you are trying to convey to him or her. Therefore, you should expect to focus considerable attention on this individual if you are anticipating support for introduced legislation or committee consideration of your issue that may result in legislation.

The relationship with committee staff members is nurtured in the same way you nurture your relationship with your congressional delegation staff. Meet with them personally and share information in a briefing document, preferably two pages or less, that encapsulates the main points of your issue of concern. The information should be relevant, describe the issue clearly, provide background and any current law associated with the issue, and include your recommendations for consideration by the committee. After your initial meeting, you should regularly supply updates and any additional information you think builds support for your issue. Take care to provide information and data that are current, rigorous, and correct. The quickest way to sour a staff relationship is providing poor or incorrect information. If any staff member, especially committee staff, requests information or input from you, be sure to provide that input as soon as possible.

Like the majority party, the minority party appoints members to leadership roles on committees. These minority party members are recognized as "ranking members" and often hold substantial sway over committee action. A ranking member's staff functions in much the same way as that of the committee chair, but often it is smaller. It is important to take the same approach to developing and maintaining relationships with minority committee staff as with majority committee staff.

Committees perform two important congressional activities. One is authorizing federal program activity; the other is appropriating funding for these programs. Every federal program must have a statutory authorization to operate and receive funding. For example, the National Institutes of Health (NIH) are authorized to operate under circumstances created in legislation called the Public Health Service Act. Reauthorizing a program can create significant change in the administration, focus, and public impact of the program. For example, members of the authorizing committees (the House Committee on Energy and Commerce and the Senate Committee on Health, Education, Labor, and Pensions) and eventually the entirety of Congress can amend the current law authorizing the operation of NIH. Program authorization or reauthorization takes place in the committee having jurisdiction over that program area. Effective advocacy for authorization of new federal programs or reauthorization of existing programs is undertaken as discussed above.

Taking Advantage of the Budget Cycle

Funding for programs is the province of the appropriations committees. Annually, funding amounts for each appropriations committee are established. These amounts are allocated from a total funding number that is usually determined by a budget target established by a budget resolution. This nonbinding legislation is developed in the House of Representatives and sent to the Senate for consideration, amendment, and passage. This nonbinding legislation is not signed by the President, but it establishes the total funding level for the federal budget.

> *You have to know the legislative territory: who makes the decisions that affect pharmacy and health care, how the system works, and how you can make an impact.*

The President does have a role in the development of the annual federal budget. Each February, the President releases a budget that reflects the priorities of the Administration for the coming year. The President's budget may or may not have a substantial impact on congressional budget development, depending on the President's political party affiliation and that of the House majority. The President's budget reflects specific interests and concerns of the individual federal agencies. Each year, starting in July, federal agencies send the Office of Management and Budget (OMB) their individual budget requests. These requested amounts are weighed against the President's priorities and may be adjusted through a series of "pass-backs" between OMB and the agency. The final result is the budget that the President submits to Congress each year at the beginning of February.

Thus, through the year as budgets are developed and allocations to appropriators are made, there are several opportunities to advocate for your interests. Advocating at the federal level includes activity in both the congressional and the administrative branches. If your issue is something that is or could be funded as a federal program, you will want to bring it to the attention of the federal agency responsible for administering the program. The agency should be made aware of your interest before its budget for the coming fiscal year is developed. This is the best opportunity to ensure that your issue will be reflected in the funding levels the agency forwards to OMB in the summer.

OMB should also be aware of your specific programmatic interest. Building upon a Presidential priority is a way to gain support for your issue and increase the chance that it will be included in the President's budget. Federal agencies, including OMB, all have Web sites that list their organizational structure and staff contact information. Using these Web-based resources is essential in federal advocacy.

Once the President's budget is submitted, congressional action takes place through the House of Representatives. Congressional budgets are divided into functional areas. It is important that the functional area that supports your issue is funded at a level that should guarantee your program's continuation and growth. Working with the House Budget Committee staff can help build awareness and support for your issue. The budget development process offers several points at which advocacy can be effective. Since both the House and Senate must agree to the budget package, there is work that can be done within both chambers. Explicit support for your issue or program can be demonstrated by the inclusion of a "sense of the House" or "sense of the Senate" in the budget legislation; this is an expression of the chamber's interest in seeing that a particular program is funded or an issue is studied throughout the session.

After the budget is determined, allocations to the appropriations committees are made. This is another point at which advocacy can be effective. The chairs of the House and Senate appropriations committees are responsible for allocating funding levels to the subcommittees. The committee chairs can be encouraged to include sufficient funding in the allocation that your program will have a good chance of being funded. Once the allocations are made, the action turns to the appropriations committees in both chambers. Traditionally the House initiates this process, but the Senate has been known to take initial action when the House is deemed unresponsive or slow in developing the funding bills. Each step of the appropriations process, from the subcommittee to the full committee and through consideration on the floor of each chamber, affords ample prospects for advocacy. Your work need not end until each chamber has come to consensus on differences between bills introduced in the respective chambers for the fiscal year funding levels.

Building Support

Once you understand the process, you will begin to appreciate the many ways in which your advocacy can have an impact. You will also recognize that advocacy is not a one-time effort. There are several points at which you can be successful, but these points can come at times when your issue is lost in the chaos of the process, or when someone else comes in with a competing issue that proves to be of greater interest to members and staff. To ensure that your issue is not lost in the shuffle, you must strengthen your position at every step of the way.

Congressional staff will rarely act on an issue that does not hold some interest to the member for whom they work. Just as rare is an issue that has never been brought to their attention. When there are competing approaches, staff will frequently expect someone to broker a consensus approach with all the stakeholders working on the issue. Creating consensus around your issue is critical; you have a powerful leveraging opportunity as a number of individuals or organizations coalesce around your issue. Bringing together all stakeholders, regardless of their position on the issue, is essential for building personal and committee staff support. Thus, to be an effective advocate, you must learn the skills of negotiation, compromise, and collaboration, as well as other leadership skills addressed in this book.

Building support for your issue will take time and should be done before you initiate congressional advocacy. It is important to have a group that can be called on to advocate for your issue in both a collective and an individual manner. Congressional activity is regularly influenced through such grassroots input. Individuals can make an impact by contacting their congressional delegation. The group as a whole can be recognized in letters to members of Congress stating that "the undersigned organizations" support the issue you are asking an office or committee to consider.

Once your stakeholders are organized and a consensus is reached, it becomes crucial that the collective message of the group is maintained by individuals. After individual members have made initial contact with their congressional delegation, further contact with committee staff will be limited to times of committee activity. Keeping communication with committee staff open is critical, but it should not be muddled by too many individuals providing the same message. The potential for overwhelming both personal and committee staff with unsolicited input is very real. Respectfully balancing your advocacy and enthusiasm for your issue with the demands on personal and committee staff will be rewarded. A valuable advocacy tool is contacting the offices of targeted members, especially those you work with regularly, to ask if they need to hear from their constituents on a particular issue. If the office is already on your side, minimizing or eliminating the office as a target can strengthen your relationship with the office. This in no way implies that grassroots advocacy is inappropriate—only that you can gain more for your issue by maintaining collegial, supportive relationships.

There are times when you have to go it alone. There will be issues around which no consensus can be reached, and times when the window of opportunity is too brief for consensus development. These times should be rare, since policy development will eventually lead to consensus development. Take the time to consider the impact of going it alone. This may be a good time to reflect on how well you have developed your relationships with staff, policy makers, stakeholders, and other interested parties. If you have done a good job in developing and maintaining relationships, calling a group of like minds to action at a moment's notice should not be a problem. Your ability to initiate change through the actions of others will be a clear indicator that you are an effective leader and advocate for your issue.

Input, Input, Input

Advocacy requires an ongoing commitment to maintaining awareness and positioning to take advantage of political timing. Successful advocacy is dependent on knowing the federal process and building support for your issue. Once you know the process, you must regularly monitor it. There are several ways to do this. Contrary to what you may believe, Congress does attempt to deal with issues relevant to the American public. You must know where your issue stands on the political agenda of both

Congress and the nation. The greater relevance your issue has to the interest and concerns of the nation, the greater is the chance that Congress will find it relevant. How will you know your issue is relevant? You must continually scan the

Advocacy is more about relationships than issues.

environment through the news media, private newsletters, and advocacy alerts from your professional organizations, and you must regularly review the actions of Congress and a host of other resources to gain a broader view of where your issue falls on political agendas.

Again, advocacy is not a one-time activity but an ongoing commitment to your issue. Scanning the environment can provide entrée to congressional staff. Keeping up with what is written on the editorial pages of leading newspapers can equip you with important information to share with staff. Letters to the editor in local newspapers from a member's district or state are recognized by staff as elements of movement of an issue within the political agenda. Bringing these to the attention of staff will strengthen your relationship. Through your willingness and ability to procure information, you will gain recognition by the staff.

The best type of information to provide to congressional staff is firsthand knowledge. Being a source of information is good, but providing staff with direct exposure to your issue builds even greater support. Congressional staff, as well as members of Congress themselves, benefit greatly from site visits and input from constituents who support your issue. If at all possible, invite members of your congressional delegation, their personal staff, and staff of committees with jurisdiction over your issue to see programs or activities that benefit from your issue. If you want more funding for the Medicare home health benefit, make sure that members and staff go on a home visit. If your issue improves individual access to care, take the member and staff to the location at which this care is provided. There is no more powerful advocacy tool than having a constituent state the importance of your issue or program.

As powerful as a site visit can be, its power will quickly wane if all the stakeholders around your issue are not part of the visit. Leaving important organizations or individuals out of the planning for a site visit by a member of Congress can lead to problems and chaos. Your need to maintain control of a site visit should be balanced with the need to have your issue seen in the best possible light. This may require you to relinquish control to others so that your message remains clear and focused to the member of Congress. Prior to the site visit all matters of engagement should be thoroughly discussed and staged, as well as what the message to the member will include. A site visit is not the time for surprises. Preparation, inclusion, and agreement are essential components that should receive attention long before your honored guest arrives.

Summary

Clearly, advocacy is more about relationships than issues. Your interest in and association with specific issues will wax and wane, but understanding the federal legislative process and maintaining relationships with key players in the process will make you an effective advocate for any issue.

Whether an issue is germane should be an important consideration as you prioritize your time and effort. Remember that this is determined both by the activity of a committee and by the political agenda of the Administration and the nation as a whole. Congress works on matters of national interest, even though those interests may benefit particular constituents, such as shipbuilders on the coasts or dairy farmers in the Northeast. The President gets elected by promising support for federal activity in any number of issue areas. It is the public that votes members of Congress and the President into office. Presenting your issue in the context of these elements of public policy making will increase the chance that it will capture the interest of the public and of elected officials.

Advocacy requires continual attention to environmental scanning, relationship maintenance, and message creation. Your messages should be crafted to give your issues or actions the most traction with a particular individual or organization (this is "spin"). As you continue your advocacy, you will need to regularly adapt your messages on the basis of your ongoing scanning. Yesterday's news is old, and your message must be presented in the context of today—and tomorrow if possible. Maintaining the relevance of your message is a difficult aspect of advocacy. Regular, frequent contact with key staff and the world around you will make it easier to create powerful messages around your issue. Too often, advocates are lulled into thinking that their professional association's annual legislative day is enough to gain federal policy makers' support for their issues. But that is not the case. Persistence, calculation, balance, and commitment are needed to keep your issue before policy makers and your message salient to the current political agenda.

Over and over again this chapter has referred to the importance of developing and maintaining relationships to build support for your issue. Successful advocacy requires you to develop and maintain relationships, both with federal policy makers and with like-minded individuals or groups that you gather in coalitions and task forces to demonstrate broad-based support for your issue. As in any relationship, being truthful, communicating directly, remaining positive, and working from a position of strength will build you greater long-term support than would the opposite behaviors. Threats, gossip, and deception should never be considered, regardless of the environment in which you are engaged. Employing strength-based advocacy will gain you quicker, more sustained support than will complaining about the past. Use positive terms to describe the strengths of your issue. New, fresh concepts challenge policy makers' minds and play to their curiosity. Try to create messages that place your issue in the context of current activity. Initiate relationships by offering assistance rather than by stating demands. Think of how you like to be approached when someone is asking you to consider changing your mind on an issue. A unique, fresh approach with strong, broad community or external support will engage the analytical and creative aspects of a policy maker's mind. You've got to know the territory.

Additional Resources

Redman E. *The Dance of Legislation.* New York: Simon & Schuster; 1973. Tells the story of the creation and passage of the National Health Service Corps Act in the 1970s.

The United States Constitution

Rules of the Senate (www.senate.gov/legislative/common/briefing/Standing_Rules_Senate.htm)

Rules of the House (www.rules.house.gov/109/text/rulesofcomm/109_rulescomm.pdf)

Lessons Learned about State Advocacy

Theresa Wells Tolle

State advocacy efforts rely on grassroots involvement. They are successful when they include many different people and groups, good communication, and a solid message. The key is to encourage pharmacists and student pharmacists to commit to advocacy, and one of the best ways to do this is through examples of how one person's idea can translate into legislative action.

Take a pharmacist we'll call Susan Snyder, who became concerned because a certain noncontrolled substance in a pain relief medication seemed to be habit forming. Susan researched the issue and consulted her colleagues, whose similar experience confirmed her fears. Susan approached her state pharmacy association leadership team to present her evidence about this serious and prevalent issue. Moved by her compelling remarks, the association officers drafted a resolution for presentation to the membership at the next state meeting. Susan presented her findings at the meeting, persuading the membership to pass a resolution that became part of the association's legislative package for the upcoming session. Association members then began advocacy through a variety of channels to convey their message to their state legislators and the general public. As a result of this advocacy, state legislators recognized that this problem could

Theresa Wells Tolle

Background

Theresa Wells Tolle, recipient of the 2004 American Pharmacists Association Good Government Pharmacist of the Year Award, is owner of Bay Street Pharmacy and Home Health Care in Roseland, Florida.

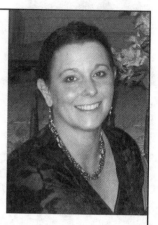

A past president of the Florida Pharmacy Association, she was instrumental in getting the Florida legislature to pass one of the nation's most comprehensive auditing standard bills for pharmacy. As a primary advocate of the bill, she helped provide insight into the policy outlined in the legislation and educated legislators on the need for this legislation.

Tolle travels regularly to Tallahassee to testify on legislation affecting pharmacists and the community. She has worked to enhance the visibility of Florida pharmacists and their valuable role in patient care through her leadership of the Florida Health Fair, an annual event in which pharmacists provide health screening for members of the state legislature and their staffs.

Tolle is a member of the Brevard County Pharmacy Association, the Florida Pharmacy Association, and the American Pharmacists Association. She received her Bachelor of Science degree in Pharmacy from the University of Florida College of Pharmacy.

Personal Statement

My interest in leadership occurred because I had a desire to be active within my profession. I wanted to be a part of a group that did community service projects, such as poison prevention programs for children. I knew these projects would bring reward and fulfillment to my regular job as a pharmacist. My interest in advocacy was piqued by a lobbyist who had worked for our state association. She took me under her wing and taught me how advocacy works at the state level.

For me, involvement was easy because I modeled what my father did. He was always active in civic and school organizations and even local county government. Many of my family members have been public servants—judges and police officers, for example. I think those influences helped me become a person who always wanted to be a doer.

I believe I have a gift for being a peacemaker. I feel that God blessed me with the ability to bring two sides together to reach consensus. I also think my personality allows people to feel comfortable approaching me and engaging in conversation. Although I don't see myself as a visionary, I do think I can lay out a road map for reaching a vision. I have tried to apply lessons I've learned about leadership in my home, at work, and in my professional circles by being more structured and self-disciplined.

It is easy to make mistakes, but I recently read that "failure is the opportunity to begin again more intelligently." I think one of the biggest mistakes is failure to be disciplined. It takes a great deal of discipline to balance one's personal, spiritual, and professional life. A mistake I have made is not reading enough and working to develop myself as a leader, but I can recommend John Maxwell's books as an excellent guide to how leaders should live their lives. I have embraced the concept that leaders cannot do everything and must learn to delegate. That is a difficult lesson for many leaders, but I am getting better at it!

cause harm to the public, and they passed a law regulating the substance.

Susan and the association declared victory and moved on to tackle other issues facing pharmacy practice. Not only had they succeeded with this particular issue, but they had laid the groundwork for future advocacy efforts. Most likely, the pharmacists who participated realize that their ideas and concerns made a difference, and they will be ready to volunteer during the next such effort.

Often, it is issues affecting their livelihood that motivate pharmacists and student pharmacists to become involved. For example, Medicaid programs are always at the top of state pharmacy associations' legislative agendas. Every year, legislators try to trim costs by making cuts in some area of the Medicaid budget, and many times pharmacy is hit hard. The cuts cause providers to choose whether they can remain a part of the Medicaid provider network and, if so, whether the pharmacy will have to make staffing changes to compensate for the cuts in reimbursement. Such monetary issues rally pharmacists to advocacy. Additional issues presenting opportunities for pharmacist advocacy at the state level relate to changes in the traditional dispensing role brought about by automation, robotic technology, central pharmacy sites, and duties of pharmacy technicians.

Coordinating Advocacy Efforts

Successful state advocacy requires coordination of various grassroots efforts, and state pharmacy associations are the logical choice to perform this role. State associations around the country go about their advocacy efforts in different ways, but the goal is to make legislators aware that an issue is important to the members of the association—and to the public. If the association sends a representative to speak with a legislator but the legislator never hears from any other pharmacist, student pharmacist, or patient, the legislator may dismiss the issue as the isolated concern of one person. Legislators will have a different perception if they receive follow-up phone calls, letters, faxes, and e-mails reinforcing the first person's message. The more consistent the message and the more persistent its advocates, the more likely it is that a legislator will vote in support of pharmacists' concerns.

In many states, several different pharmacy associations represent various practice settings, such as health-system pharmacists, consultant pharmacists, and independent or community pharmacists. Occasionally, one association's advocacy might focus on a specific practice setting and might be in conflict with the legislative priorities of the other state associations. It is important that all pharmacy organizations attempt to work together from the outset. They should meet together, share legislative priorities, find common ground, and even discuss their differences and how they should proceed. As I will discuss later, a unified message is crucial.

Building Relationships

At the state level as at the national level, the most effective way to achieve ongoing legislative support is through personal relationships with individual representatives and senators. These relationships can develop because the legislator is your patient or neighbor, attends your church, belongs to your club, or is related to you, or just because you take time to visit his or her office. Through your regular visits, both to the legislator's home district office and to the state capital during the legislative session, the legislator becomes comfortable with you and will call on you when an issue specific to pharmacy arises.

You can also develop such a relationship by volunteering to work on a legislator's campaign. There are numerous opportunities, such as answering the phone at the campaign office, initiating phone calls, walking door to door, holding a sign, or organizing a fundraiser. Every pharmacist and student pharmacist should find a few hours to donate to the candidates of their choice. Legislators do not quickly forget people who work side by side with them.

Should We Use Professional Lobbyists?

State associations vary in their financial resources and level of volunteer commitment to organizing advocacy efforts. Several state associations have hired an executive or staff member who is primarily responsible for directing advocacy strategies. Across the country, the staffing of pharmacy associations ranges from one part-time staff member to a staff of more than 30, and the larger associations can dedicate more staff resources to advocacy. Some associations have legislative councils or committees that develop the agenda for the session and solicit volunteers from the membership to be the "legs" of the advocacy effort. Many associations have hired lobbyists or lobbying firms that specialize in health care and understand the issues relevant to pharmacy.

Lobbyists can be very effective in helping an organization establish relationships with the right people. Legislators get to know the lobbyist, who is in their office often discussing issues, working to fine-tune legislation, and asking them to sponsor or co-sponsor legislation. The legislator becomes comfortable picking up the phone and calling the lobbyist about any issue related to pharmacy before voting. Associations have found that another effective role of the lobbyist is to take the pulse of the legislature and keep the association members and leadership informed about what is happening. A good lobbyist will anticipate key issues before they arise, or at least identify them as soon as they surface. The lobbyist will report on issues to the membership and provide direction on effective communication with the legislators.

In considering a lobbying firm, the association must evaluate its financial resources. Some states have income streams to support such efforts, while others do not. Each state association must determine what best suits its needs and resources. The Florida Pharmacy Association (FPA), for example, has had great success using a lobbying firm for many years.

A lobbyist can help an association develop a grassroots network of key pharmacists and student pharmacists in the state who are politically active or who have a relationship with their state representative or senator or that person's staff. A mechanism is needed for quickly communicating with key members of the network (e.g., by telephone, fax, e-mail, or a combination). During the legislative session in particular, issues arise that may necessitate a turnaround time of a few hours. It is imperative to have a system for reaching key members who will contact their legislators and spread the word to colleagues who will do the same. Regardless of the size and financial resources of an association, this type of grassroots effort can work. It is critical, however, that the message to be communicated to legislators is clearly conveyed to the grassroots network and that members of the network deliver the message consistently.

Using Technology

Many state and national associations use Internet-based technology to help them communicate with their members, provide members an easy way to identify and contact their legislators, and track all of the contacts made. For example, FPA uses Capwiz·XC (www.capitoladvantage.com/capwiz/qt/intro.html), an innovative government relations research tool that helps organizations effectively communicate with state and federal elected officials and increase member participation in advocacy. Because of its cost, this tool may not be ideal for every association. However, it is extremely helpful for getting a message out to interested parties quickly, controlling the consistency of the message that goes out, assisting pharmacists and student pharmacists in locating all of their legislators (state and national), and finally providing a report to the association about how many contacts have been made through the site. This last function is particularly helpful because it is good to know how many times a particular legislator has heard a message, especially when the legislator maintains that he or she has not heard from pharmacists at all. With Capwiz·XC or a similar program, associations can have those numbers with just a few keystrokes. It may even help the association to gently remind the legislator to check his or her messages again!

Political Action Committees and Fundraising

Politicians will tell you that, like it or not, it takes money to get into office. Candidates need to raise money to run for office, and they rely on financial contributions by their constituents and supporters. In addition, with our two-party government system, legislators are often seeking to raise money to support other candidates of their party or help move the party agenda forward.

As part of advocacy, it is important to consider financial contributions to legislative members who are "friends" of pharmacy. This can take the form of funds from individual pharmacists, business owners, or other pharmacy partners. It is important for constituent pharmacists and student pharmacists to personally contribute as often as possible, since this helps

Successful state advocacy requires coordination of various grassroots efforts, and state pharmacy associations are the logical choice to perform this role.

develop a personal relationship with the legislator or candidate.

A more effective way to contribute might be through a political action committee (PAC). State laws differ in regard to specific dollar limits on donations to or from a PAC, and it is important to understand your state's law if a PAC is being considered. The state division of elections governs these committees. PACs can accumulate a great deal of money, which is why they are so effective. It is best to develop a strategy before each legislative session or election campaign concerning the number of donations the PAC should be giving and the dollar amount for each donation. That allows the PAC to set a goal for fundraising. It is also important to note that many states restrict the timing of contributions. For example, in Florida PACs cannot donate any money to legislators during a legislative session.

Fundraising can be handled in many ways, including solicitation through the annual dues statement, personal letters, luncheons, raffles, or whatever is legal. Independent pharmacy owners are usually very involved in PAC donations because their businesses can be greatly affected by legislative changes. Typically, this is an area where the lobbyist has great influence over who should receive contributions and the strategy for giving those contributions.

Think Success

State advocacy requires a lot of work, but I have found it to be extremely rewarding. I often use the letters of "success" to summarize the important elements of state advocacy:

S: Solidify the message of the issue that is being advocated. The issue needs to be something that is worth a legislator's time. To the extent possible, it is best to focus on the effect it will have on patient care.

U: Understanding of the issues by pharmacists and student pharmacists, and by legislators and their staffers, must be ensured. If an issue is not well presented, it will be more difficult to get buy-in and sponsors for the legislation.

C: Communication cannot be overemphasized. Advocacy is extremely dependent on communication to the grassroots and then from the grassroots back to legislators. Remember that you are a patient advocate and represent a large number of voting constituents. Don't be afraid to get patients involved in legislative advocacy. They can be very effective, especially in large numbers.

C: Consistency of the message is especially important when there are numerous pharmacy groups within a state and their agendas are not the same. Nothing kills an issue quicker than for legislators to receive mixed messages from within the same profession. The legislators do not understand that different practice settings may be represented, and they may perceive that pharmacy is not together on the issue.

E: Everyone should participate. Associations should strive to involve all of their members. A loud, united voice goes further than a few lone voices speaking over and over.

S: Solicit funds for PACs. Money talks, especially in the political world. It is very important to support legislators who have been pharmacy-friendly. A friend in the legislature can sometimes be difficult to find, especially if there are no pharmacists serving as representatives or senators.

S: Support pharmacist candidates. States should be constantly building a pipeline of pharmacists who are interested in public service at any level. No one has a pharmacist's unique perspective on the profession, and having a pharmacist in the legislature is particularly helpful. Many states have one or more pharmacists in their statehouses and numerous others serving at all levels of government.

STATUTE TO REGULATION: A CONTINUUM OF AUTHORITY

Raymond C. Love

I n the early 1980s, I was a young clinical pharmacist working in a state-operated psychiatric facility. I was appalled to see inpatients who sat untreated in the facility for months or years. For the most part, they were out of touch with reality and deteriorating psychiatrically, emotionally, and sometimes physically. Why did these individuals remain untreated? Because state laws regarding involuntary commitment to a psychiatric facility were distinct and unrelated to the laws regarding competency. We could not treat those patients without their consent, even though we could keep them in a hospital against their will. If we treated them against their will, we would be violating their rights. I began to argue repeatedly that we were also violating their rights by not helping them.

Dr. Robert Grooms, the facility superintendent, encouraged me to submit my concern to a newly developed statewide quality assurance program. He assured me that the new system was set up in such a manner that concerns would be elevated through the facility and state mental health system until they reached a level with the authority to address them. After several months, I was summoned to a meeting with Assistant Secretary of Health and Mental Hygiene Dr. Stanley Platman, who greeted me and

101

Raymond C. Love

Background

Raymond C. Love is Vice-Chair of the Department of Pharmacy Practice and Science at the University of Maryland School of Pharmacy. He also serves as director of the school's mental health program, overseeing pharmacy services in the state of Maryland's psychiatric facilities. Love served as a member of the Maryland Board of Pharmacy for 8 years, chairing the Pharmacy Practice Committee and holding the office of treasurer of the board. He has been an active member of the legislative committees of state pharmacy associations and represents the College of Psychiatric and Neurologic Pharmacists on the Pharmacist Provider Coalition, a group of seven national pharmacy organizations that advocates for improved care by allowing Medicare patients access to the expertise of pharmacists and better integrating pharmacists into the health care team.

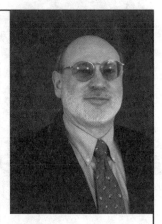

Personal Statement

It is often difficult to advocate for oneself or one's peers without sounding self-serving. One lesson I have learned is that you need to know who has the most influence over the persons to whom you direct your advocacy efforts. Legislators often want to hear from other professionals and voters. The words of a patient who supports your position ring louder than the voices of a dozen professionals. When a matter treads on professional turf boundaries, the words of members of the public can make the positions of professionals seem petty and self-serving.

The higher one moves in government or in any large organization, the greater is the role that politics plays in any decision. Politics trumps rationality, financial feasibility, ethics, and even the interests of the public. In one of my early experiences, I was amazed that a legislator acted contrary to my logically developed, painstakingly articulated position—after telling me she would vote for it. Some years later, I confronted the legislator, who confessed that, in a horse trade, she had cast a vote opposing what she knew to be correct in order to garner support from another legislator for her pet project.

Integrating advocacy into my professional life is a challenge because advocacy and leadership both take time. It is not feasible to partake of every leadership opportunity and advocate for every cause. We must choose the opportunities that mean the most. And with e-mail, fax, and telephones, we can be part-time advocates without the greater time commitment of face-to-face interaction. A phone call following an e-mail to emphasize important points can have a dramatic impact with a minimal time commitment.

It is difficult to stay informed about everything that goes on. State and national pharmacy organizations, trade groups, and even employers commit resources to keeping tabs on Congress, legislative agencies, and regulatory bodies. They use their list servers, Web pages, and other resources to help keep members and employees informed and to occasionally rally the troops. To take advantage of these resources, all you need to do is join, sign up, or make known your desire to be included.

introduced me to a variety of administrators, academics, and assistant attorneys general. They informed me that my concern was timely. Before I knew it, I was traveling 300 miles back and forth every 2 weeks from my facility in Cumberland, Maryland, to the state offices in Baltimore to work on the issue.

After months of work, we had crafted a piece of legislation that would create clinical review panels to hear the concerns of patients and the clinicians responsible for treating them. The bill would allow short involuntary trials of treatment against the patient's will for those who had no possibility of discharge from the state's custody. If the patient failed to respond or had untoward side effects, the trials would be stopped. Patients who responded favorably would be asked if they had changed their minds and wanted to consent to continued treatment. The bill was submitted to the state legislature by the executive branch and was passed. Almost miraculously, most of the patients who underwent the clinical review panel process responded to medication, later consented to treatment, and eventually were discharged. These patients with severe psychiatric disorders, who were too paranoid to consent or who might have had a previous bad experience with medication, were no longer destined to wallow indefinitely in inpatient facilities.

I not only learned that one individual could make a difference; I learned that one person can make a significant impact by challenging the status quo.

From Statute to Regulation

An old German proverb states that "the devil is in the details." The public hears debates about new laws (statutes) passed by Congress or a state legislature; the laws may be passed to provide funding, establish programs, provide structure, resolve disputes, provide opportunities, or put in place new limits. But laws are often concepts that lack sufficient detail for implementation. Does Congress worry about the speed with which pharmacists are reimbursed when it passes a program like the Medicare Part D benefit? Does a state legislature worry about how many continuing-education credits pharmacists need in the area of

> *Each health professional has an important role to play in the process of shaping health care through legislation and regulation. The health professional is responsible for continually educating decision makers about the needs of the profession and how the system can better serve the public.*

pharmacy law or pain management? Probably not. So how are those details determined?

Although legislative bodies can put into a statute as much detail as they want, they generally refrain from doing so. They usually delegate specifics to departments (e.g., department of health), agencies (e.g., insurance commission), or boards (e.g., board of pharmacy, board of regents). These government entities are then charged with proposing regulations that implement the law. It is here that the details are worked out.

For instance, most states have laws that either charge a pharmacy with having "adequate" security or charge the board of pharmacy with developing regulations for the operation of pharmacies in a manner that promotes the public health and safety. A board of pharmacy may propose regulations concerning what types of individuals can be behind a pharmacy prescription counter, whether anyone can enter a pharmacy without a pharmacist present, how prescription medications and controlled substances must be stored, whether alarm systems are necessary, and so on.

State laws require that applicants for pharmacist licensure pass an examination or examinations approved by the board of pharmacy. However, the specific examination (North American Pharmacist Licensure Examination [NAPLEX]), examinations (NAPLEX and Multistate Pharmacy Jurisprudence Examination [MPJE]), or criteria for the examinations are usually identified in regulations. By the same token, changing existing regulations does not require legislative action. For years, many states required licensure applicants to take a compounding practical examination. The decision to eliminate this examination in Maryland was quite controversial. However, eliminating the exam took nothing more than the passage of a regulation by the board of pharmacy.

Often, a board of pharmacy or other state agency decides that it needs to address an area not specifically designated in the law. For many years, the existence of pharmacy technicians and pharmacy assistants was ignored by state law in Maryland. Almost every pharmacy employs technicians and other nonpharmacists who have access to drugs and sensitive patient information and who play vital roles in the prescription process and pharmacy operations. The Maryland Board of Pharmacy was challenged by a legislator who wanted to ensure that someone had jurisdiction over the training and activities of these individuals. However, these individuals could not legally exist under state law. According to state law, the activities performed by these nonpharmacists could be carried out only by pharmacists. Because the law did not recognize these individuals, the board had no statutory authority over them and thus could not regulate them. What could the board of pharmacy do?

There was a great debate over whether the board of pharmacy should propose to the state legislature a bill recognizing pharmacy technicians. Some pharmacists were concerned about being replaced by technicians. Others were concerned about the requirements for becoming a technician and how they might affect existing technicians and future recruitment of technicians. Meanwhile, the questions from legislators continued, and the board had to act.

Finally, the board realized the solution. It could regulate pharmacy permit holders (pharmacy owners), pharmacy operations, and pharmacists under its statutory mandate. Therefore, it could decide how one must train and supervise and what one could delegate to those employed in the pharmacy. Using these existing laws as a reason to act, the board proposed and the state adopted regulations regarding the use of "nonlicensed personnel" in pharmacies. Eventually, the legislature and the board recognized that it was in the state's best interest to be able to directly regulate technicians rather than just the pharmacists who supervise them, the pharmacies in which they work, and the permit holders who hire them. For this reason, the Maryland legislature changed the pharmacy practice act (a statute) to recognize pharmacy technicians and charged the board of pharmacy with regulating them.

From Proposed to Adopted

Administrative entities are charged with proposing regulations, which are powerful rules. Violation of a regulation can result in penalties and loss of rights or privileges. In most states, if you violate a motor vehicle administration regulation, you are subject to fines and perhaps even imprisonment. Because they have such important ramifications, regulations usually must go through a series of reviews before they take effect.

Either during development or after they are passed by a board of pharmacy or other state agency, regulations are reviewed for legal sufficiency by a staff attorney or an assistant attorney general. This review might find that the regulation conflicts with an existing statute or regulation (federal or state), is unclear, was proposed without adequate statutory authority, violates an inherent legal right, or has some other legal deficiency. If the regulation is found to be legally sufficient, it is passed on to the next level.

In most cases, regulations are then reviewed by some higher executive branch entity such as a cabinet-level appointee (e.g., secretary of health), head of an agency (e.g., federal Occupational Safety and Health Administration), or representative of the state governor. This individual then authorizes disclosure of the pending regulation to the public. The federal government publishes the *Federal Register* to inform interested parties of proposed regulations. Most states maintain similar state registers (e.g., *The Texas Register, The Maryland Register, The Virginia Register of Regulations*), which are published at regular intervals. The registers list the proposed regulations, the time interval during which comments will be accepted, and the address to which comments should be directed.

After publication in the register, the process may vary according to the jurisdiction (specific state or federal), the agency, and the urgency of the regulation. For instance, in the wake of Hurricane Katrina, some states passed emergency regulations dealing with price gouging that required no comment period and went into effect immediately. In most cases, comments are reviewed by those who initially proposed the regulations. The reviewers may ignore some comments, reply to those offering comments, alter the regulation in a nonsubstantive manner (correct grammar or unclear wording), or make substantive changes in the proposed regulation. In most cases, regulations that undergo substantive modifications must be republished for another comment period.

Once a regulation has been published and the comments addressed, it is generally republished with an "effective" date on which it has the force of law. Most states have an established process that allows a special legislative review committee a veto over problematic or controversial regulations.

Implementation

The adoption of a regulation does not end the process. Next, the regulation must be implemented. In the case of a board of pharmacy, this may involve simple steps such as notifying pharmacists or pharmacy permit holders, more complex actions such as changing applications and application processes, or extensive development of new systems to implement programs such as registration of pharmacy technicians.

Sometimes legislatures try to satisfy a variety of interested parties by agreeing to compromises. When a board of pharmacy or other agency tries to implement a statute that contains too many compromises, problems can ensue. For example, when the Maryland legislature passed the state's collaborative drug therapy management bill, compromises were made to prevent opposition by the state medical society. The statute required multiple documents, including a physician–pharmacist agreement, a therapy management contract with the physician, and patient and drug therapy protocols. Furthermore, the board of physicians and board of pharmacy were jointly charged with implementation of the program; therefore, both boards were charged with developing regulations for implementation. Obviously, this was a matter of highest importance to the board of pharmacy, so it took the lead. Not only did it have to propose the regulations, but the board of pharmacy then had to explain and "sell" them to the board of physicians. The difficulty in drafting regulations and then explaining them was confounded by the three-document system incorporated to get the bill passed; the legislation required that each agreement have the approval of both the pharmacy and physician boards. An agreement eventually was reached, but the complexity of the process and the specifics prescribed by the legislature have slowed the progress of collaborative drug therapy management in Maryland.

> *I learned that one person can make a significant impact by challenging the status quo.*

Compromise can necessitate working with the opposition in the implementation process. For example, pharmacists in Maryland initially sought the privilege to administer medication instead of seeking only the ability to immunize. The pharmacy community reasoned that pharmacists are responsible for teaching patients and family members to administer liquid, ophthalmic, inhaled, otic, and topical preparations. They teach those with diabetes, allergies, and other disorders how to self-administer medications. Home infusion and hospital pharmacists teach nurses how to administer medication, operate pumps, and clear lines. Why shouldn't pharmacists be allowed to administer medications?

The broad application of pharmacist medication administration was met with insurmountable opposition by nurses. One nurse legislator spoke in support of pharmacists on the issue of collaborative drug therapy management, but she made it clear that medication administration was the sole purview of nurses. After several legislative failures, pharmacists finally were able to win the ability to immunize, but this authority was limited to influenza vaccination only.

The final law required the boards of nursing and physicians to collaborate with the board of pharmacy in the development of immunization regulations, and the board of nursing did not prove to be the most willing partner in the process. The physician and pharmacy boards quickly agreed that the pharmacist needed to be able to administer emergency medication in the event of an allergic reaction after influenza vaccine administration, but the board of nursing took the position that the administration of agents other than influenza vaccine by pharmacists was not legal. Eventually, the regulations succeeded, thanks to behind-the-scenes efforts by members of the boards who worked together daily in the real (as opposed to the regulatory) world.

Regulations Are Not Forever

Once a law is passed, it is "on the books" forever, unless it is repealed by an act of a legislature or contains a clause that causes it to become invalid on a certain date. The life of regulations varies and may be self-limiting. Some regulations state that they will expire on a specific date. In addition, many states limit the period during which an emergency regulation can be effective. It is common to limit an emergency regulation to a period sufficient to propose and adopt a permanent regulation, or to 180 days.

Sometimes, statutes and regulations are subject to "sunset" provisions. These are an automatic way of forcing the legislature or administrative entities to periodically review laws and regulations. Boards of pharmacy in many states have a regular schedule for reviewing regulations in their purview. If the board does not reapprove these regulations on schedule (or request an extension), they expire after their "sunset" date.

Even agencies themselves may be subject to "sunsetting." Several years ago, the Maryland General Assembly took issue with the Maryland Board of Medical Examiners and failed to renew the statute that would keep the board operational. The former board faded from existence, to be replaced by a Board of Physicians that had a new membership.

Find Allies, Compromise Carefully

As the health care system changes and pharmacists find innovative ways to serve the public, the potential for treading on the turf of other professions will increase. In both the proposal of legislation and the drafting of regulations, pharmacy will need to compromise. However, the profession must be sure not to give away too much. We should heed the maxim "Compromise now; pay later!" A statute or regulation that will not work or that produces intolerable consequences is not a victory. Society does not need a "cure that is worse than the disease."

One key to success in the emerging interprofessional environment of regulation is finding allies in other professions who will advocate for pharmacy before their professional boards without appearing to be self-serving. A board of nursing is more likely to hear a message coming from a nurse than one delivered by a pharmacist. Given the role of the physician in health care, a physician ally becomes an effective advocate before multiple agencies and professional boards. Professional boards are charged with protecting and furthering the health and safety of the public. Thus, most have public members who represent the needs of the common citizen without entangling conflicts of interest. These board members are often the most effective at influencing administrative agencies and legislatures.

Legislators and government officials are also effective allies in advancing or opposing regulations and legislation. One of the most influential advancements in pharmacy reimbursement in Maryland was championed by a well-meaning legislator who could influence other legislators and governmental entities.

Stay Vigilant, Read the Fine Print, Protect the Public

Each health professional has an important role to play in the process of shaping health care through legislation and regulation. The health professional is responsible for continually educating decision makers about the needs of the profession and how the system can better serve the public. The health professional is also responsible for staying vigilant about emerging issues, legislation, and regulation. Depending on professional organizations may not be sufficient.

Consider the following example. A recent bill was proposed in a state legislature to regulate pharmacy benefit managers (PBMs). The bill permitted PBMs to make substitutions that resulted in financial savings that were passed on to the purchaser. This seemed like a noble provision to the staff member who wrote the bill, the legislator who sponsored it, the pharmacy association that supported it, and even the PBMs that were trying to hold down costs. They all assumed that the provision in question dealt with generic substitutions.

Fortunately, the bill was sent to an outside pharmacist reviewer for comment. The reviewer asked what the intent of the bill was and why certain language was used that was ambiguous to pharmacists. The reviewer discovered that the ambiguous language in the bill would have inadvertently given PBMs the power to prescribe. The bill was quickly tabled and died in the legislative committee. We should never underestimate the importance of asking for clarification or trying to understand why legislation and regulations are being proposed. Legislative language and regulatory verbiage mean different things to the lawyers who draft them and the health professionals who must live with them.

When signing a contract, it is always important to read the fine print. In working on regulations and legislation, reading the fine print is crucial. The language is written by lawyers but implemented by health professionals. The two groups use language differently and make different assumptions. If a health professional and a lawyer get different meanings from the same language, society loses.

Boards of pharmacy and other administrative agencies that propose laws and regulations are charged with protecting and advocating for the interests of the public. Often, the motives of these entities are consistent with the needs of the profession, but sometimes they are not. Controversies arise when an administrative entity seems to be serving a profession or business interest instead of the public. Some of pharmacy's greatest victories have come when the profession has advocated a position that is best for the public, rather than what is best for pharmacy.

Elements of Effective Lobbying

Carriann E. Richey

I n 1994, I completed my bachelor's degree in biology. I interviewed with pharmaceutical companies, research facilities, and medical laboratories. However, it seemed that my lack of a master's degree and the large number of biology graduates in the job market were working to my disadvantage. I decided to interview at a local health insurance company where I had worked as a copy and file clerk in the summers. There I applied for a new legislative analyst position that was created when the government relations department restructured to better respond to issues surrounding health care reform. Toward the end of the interview, I said that although I needed this job, I wasn't really into politics. The interviewer responded, "Name one part of your life that isn't affected by politics." My reaction was a blank stare, some blinking, and a head scratch. To my amazement, I was offered that position the following week, and within a few months I was lobbying at the state level.

I still told myself that I'd taken the job to improve my communication skills, but inevitably I learned a great deal about the political process, insurance, and health care. One of my early mistakes was underestimating the role of last-minute language changes in the legislative process. We were working very hard

Carriann E. Richey
Background

Carriann Richey is Director of Postgraduate Education and Assistant Professor of Pharmacy Practice at Butler University. As Director of the Office of Postgraduate Education, Richey serves as an Accreditation Council for Pharmacy Education continuing-education provider, with an interest in continuous professional development. Her academic responsibilities include teaching Ethics in Health Care and Delivery of Health Care. She is a co-advisor for the pharmacy leadership society Phi Lambda Sigma and an active member of the Indiana Pharmacists Alliance.

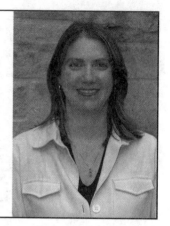

on a bill concerning medical savings accounts and were on target for a successful vote after 6 months of face-to-face conversations, trips, meetings, and dinners. Unfortunately, legislators altered the language at the last minute, trading language that was unacceptable to us for language in another bill that improved school busing. I sat there with my mouth open. After all our work, we could not compete with images of children waiting in the cold for the bus.

While working as a lobbyist, I attended a lecture by the dean of Butler University College of Pharmacy and Health Sciences. The lecture highlighted recent legislative challenges associated with pharmacy and physician assistant practice in Indiana. Through my involvement with this legislation I was exposed to pharmacy, and I decided to return to school for a pharmacy degree. Although I enjoyed my pharmacy studies, politics remained an important component of my life. Whether I liked it or hated it, I knew I had to live with politics. This chapter summarizes lessons I have learned through my experiences as an educator and a lobbyist.

Recently, as I attended our state pharmacy legislative day, I wondered what motivated 50 pharmacists (out of more than 6,000 registered in the state) to attend the event. Certainly, many were there to discuss Medicare and Medicaid problems with legislators. But more important, they knew that they had to speak for themselves, that no one else was going to act for them, and that health care reform seemed to have forgotten the pharmacist. And they believed in the future of the profession. Some came with youthful optimism and inquiry; others came out of wisdom and necessity. Regardless of their past experiences, they came because they cared. They cared about their own practice and their patients. They cared enough to stand up and fight.

Advocacy

Out of this passion comes advocacy, which takes many forms. It may be speaking, writing, or acting in support of a personal interest. Pharmacists serve as advocates by explaining the profession, our specific skill sets and abilities, and the many roles of pharmacists. They write and publish pharmacists' success stories. They demonstrate how pharmacists' efforts enhance patients' outcomes, satisfaction, and quality of life. In all these ways, pharmacists are advocates for the profession.

According to one source, "Advocacy is about saying to decision makers, potential partners, funders, [or] any stakeholder, 'Your agenda will be greatly assisted by what we have to offer.' Advocacy is about getting support from those who are in a position to help you."[1] Pharmacists' advocacy may be directed toward internal contacts such as management or external clients such as customers, patients, or individuals of influence. Pharmacists participate in advocacy through membership in local and national professional organizations, which in turn acknowledge, highlight, and recognize the accomplishments of their members.

Structured Lobbying

In addition to advocacy, most professional organizations engage in more structured lobbying, involving both volunteer and paid efforts. Like advocacy, lobbying involves education and information sharing. But lobbying aims to more directly influence legislation and voting behavior. Volunteer lobbying generally involves direct advocacy to politicians and lawmakers. The activities of a lobbyist may include meeting directly with legislators and their staff, testifying, attending social events, advertising, and grassroots polling. Political action groups, committees, and coalitions raise funds to support lobbying activities and campaign contributions; these groups have greatly increased in popularity since the 1980s.

Paid lobbying involves additional relationship building and a more consistent, directed effort. Paid lobbyists can devote more time and energy to ensuring success. A growing number of interest groups are benefiting from the advocacy of paid lobbyists, and organizations that rely on volunteer lobbying alone may find it difficult to succeed. Paid lobbyists are regulated by lobbying laws and must register their activities. To qualify as a lobbyist for federal purposes, an individual must be employed or retained by a client for financial or other compensation.

Several trends support the increase in health care lobbying:[2]

1. Congress earmarks more and more money each year for health care projects.
2. Lobbyists are increasingly relied upon as expert consultants on the economics of health care policy.
3. Lobbyists have increased influence on political campaigns through the use of pollsters and advertising to sway the public.
4. Lobbying groups may focus on smaller groups of legislators.
5. Health care accounts for more than 15% of the nation's economy.

The worst situation for any special interest group is invisibility. Pharmacists must remember that any political action, whether through advocacy or lobbying, can be beneficial.

Checks on Lobbying

Although most lobbying efforts do not involve unethical behavior, the media are quick to publicize examples of such behavior. Coverage of inappropriate behavior by politicians sells newspapers and magazines. Lobbying and special interest campaigning are often viewed with distrust by the general public, but political scientists have found little evidence to support this perspective.[3]

Studies have demonstrated few conclusive links between campaign or lobbying efforts and actual patterns of influence. Although such patterns or individual instances may exist, their impact is difficult to determine, particularly when groups claim freedom from any outside source.

In response to negative views of lobbying, the formation of ethics review committees has grown in popularity. These committees scrutinize details of money exchange and activity reports. States may enact ethics legislation designed to "rein in the power of lobbyists," as Tennessee Governor Phil Bredesen said upon signing his state's ethics bill into law.[4] Such laws have prompted lobbyists to officially identify themselves. For example, during the year following passage of the federal Lobbying Disclosure Act, the number of new organizations and individuals registering as lobbyists tripled from the previous year. Ten years later, the total number of registered lobbyists had almost doubled.[5]

Although some may consider lobbying in itself a profession, others may disagree.[6] Professionalism is more than individual practitioners doing their jobs well. A profession involves ethics, norms, values, and organization. Thus, various elements of society have developed standards for lobbying. For example, legislation has been passed to scrutinize lobbying efforts and establish acceptable behaviors, such as reporting sources of financial payment for lobbying activities, registering lobbying activity, monitoring postemployment behavior, and establishing professional responsibilities for legislators or attorneys. At the federal level, both the House of Representatives and the Senate have adopted formal codes of conduct and have formed standing committees to interpret rules and investigate charges of misconduct.

Lobbying Commandments

Wolpe[7] has suggested five "commandments" to help lobbyists manage ethical conflict:

1. **Tell the truth.** Lobbying is an educational process. Just as physicians may use pharmacists as their medication experts, legislators use lobbyists as their information sources. To maintain credibility, lobbyists must convey accurate information.

Wolpe refers to lobbying as "the political management of information." Failure to disclose important information can be just as detrimental as providing inaccurate information. The challenge for lobbyists is to know when to share information, understand how to share it, and appraise the political environment surrounding each issue. Lobbyists' fundamental purpose is to encourage and influence legislators to vote and support issues. The wrong information in the legislator's pocket benefits no one.

2. **Never promise more than you can deliver.** Promises made by lobbyists to legislators may include the votes of others, committee outcomes, or grassroots support. When a lobbyist promises the votes of other legislators, a legislator has confidence that with this support his or her own vote is more likely to count. The committee level is where much of the detailed work on legislation takes place; success can depend on the work done here. Whether a legislator has initiated certain legislation or has a vested interest in it, the ability of a lobbyist to ensure a successful outcome strengthens the relationship between the legislator and the group represented by the lobbyist. Finally, grassroots support suggests public and constituent backing. Positive results in all of these areas lead to happy constituents and eventual re-election. Success in each area requires time, energy, and presence. Again, the key for the lobbyist is veracity. Assessing workload and conflicts of interest among multiple clients and having a specific plan can guide both the paid and the volunteer lobbyist.

3. **Know how to listen so that you accurately understand what you are hearing.** The language of political decision making and social politeness can make lobbying a tricky proposition. Wolpe gives examples of phrases that may be construed to indicate commitment but are better interpreted as simply supportive: "I believe you have a good case" and "I think we should do something about this." Legislators are from different backgrounds, and good relationship building improves success in communication. Even when legislators are committed, changes in language during the legislative process may require a choice between two interests or a compromise between peers for support. For example, if

a legislator is interested both in Medicaid reimbursement rates and in efforts to improve school test scores, the legislator may have to compromise on improving reimbursement rates in order to gain peer support for school funding to improve test scores. The legislator may weigh the success of the Medicaid reimbursement effort and determine that it is better to win on one count than to fail on two. The legislator may believe that the political arrangements this year will lead to improved success next year, but may still change his or her mind on the basis of final testimony.

4. **Remember that staff is there to be worked with, not circumvented.** Each legislator has staff members who provide guidance and information. Staff are likely to understand the language of their leaders and be aware of their mannerisms, behaviors, preferences, and political alignments. Wolpe notes that "winning the confidence of staff—and maintaining it thereafter—is a prerequisite to an ongoing, successful political relationship with any political office." Federal legislators typically have several staff members in each office. The administrative assistant fills the role of office manager and is involved in all key political decisions. Legislative assistants support committee work and have responsibilities for different issues; they provide supporting information for their office as well as for the chairs of assigned committees. A personal secretary handles the legislator's travel, appointments, and schedule. Face time with the legislator may seem of highest priority, but neglecting the staff will prove detrimental in the end. This is analogous to pharmacists who focus on physician detailing and forget that office receptionists and nurses fulfill important roles, including managing the physician's appointment schedule.

5. **Spring no surprises.** At times, lobbyists must deliver negative reports to their legislators, such as changes in public opinion, emergence of peer conflicts, or unfavorable coverage in the media. Immediately disclosing this information to legislators is crucial. A lobbyist who provides up-to-date information will gain credibility and support with legislators. The lobbyist may also provide timely responses and counterarguments.

Doing the Homework

Lobbyists, paid or unpaid, should approach their work with detailed strategic planning. This includes preparing ahead of time for each lobbying visit and being able to quickly and directly state the purpose and intended outcome at the start of each visit. To provide details that cannot be covered in a short visit, a clear, concise, and persuasive summary can be left with the staff or legislator. The material should directly relate to the bill under consideration. An experienced lobbyist will learn the legislator's schedule and avoid times when he or she might be busy preparing for other events of the day.

Relationships are very important to successful lobbying, and building relationships involves knowing the players' concerns and preferences and using this knowledge in your approach. Lobbyists who arm themselves with such information know where to find allies when they need them. Allies, either within the legislature or outside, increase the lobbyist's scope of influence. Lobbyists should support the relationships they build by being readily available but not monopolizing staff and member time.

Legislators do most of their hands-on work in committees. Successful lobbyists need to know the makeup, the chair, and the disposition of committees relevant to their issue. For example, a committee might be considering various pieces of legislation on a topic, whose language varies in both major and minor ways. Familiarity with the committee would enable the lobbyist and legislator to anticipate the language differences on which to focus and the likelihood that their language will be accepted.

A legislator's goals are public benefit and re-election. Lobbyists must know the public policy rationale for an issue and use it to support their statements and facts and refute those of their adversaries. Preparing a sheet that lists potential objections, identifies the objecting individuals or groups, and explains their reasoning will prevent surprises and facilitate counterarguments. For example, if the goal is gaining approval for collaborative practice in a state that does not yet allow this for pharmacists, the list of objections might include concerns that the number of individuals involved in a patient's care should be limited and that pharmacists in some settings do not have enough information to practice at this level. With the objections identified, it is possible to determine which groups are involved, such as physician practice groups, nurse practitioners, or physician assistants. With this information at hand, the lobbyist can meet with those groups, focus on their reasoning, and present counter-arguments—which in this case might involve a discussion of mechanisms pharmacists use to retrieve patient

Like advocacy, lobbying involves education and information sharing. But lobbying aims to more directly influence legislation and voting behavior.

information or of pharmacists' frequent contact with patients and ability to have a positive impact on care. Data and studies can be used to support the counterarguments.

An advantage of using paid lobbyists is their extensive experience with the legislative process. Their knowledge of the fine points of the rules of procedure and the art of compromise are most valuable in highly controversial and public debates. They understand the process of amendments, committee activity, deliberation, and timing, and they have perspective on both sides of an issue.

Electronic Access

A discussion of lobbying and advocacy would not be complete without reference to electronic communication via the Internet. By the end of 2001, an estimated 1 million e-mail messages were sent to Congress each day, in addition to the hundreds of thousands of pieces of mail, phone calls, and faxes.[8] (Congress has a central telephone and e-mail exchange and a postal address.) Individual legislators manage their Web sites as they wish. Committees and leadership offices also maintain Web sites, the use of which depends on the type of business conducted and the likelihood of a technologically proficient audience. Filters for ZIP codes or key words are used to automatically identify e-mail from the legislator's district or state.

Those involved in direct advocacy and unpaid lobbying rely heavily on electronic communication. Grassroots lobbying efforts and special interest groups may use electronic alerts to ask members to electronically contact their senator or representative. This may or may not be effective, depending on the target legislator, office, or committee. For a paid lobbyist, the Internet is not the primary means of communication; face-to-face meetings, with two-way communication, are still preferable. The Internet gives citizens access to information about their legislators, committees, and voting results more quickly than ever before. Advocates and lobbyists can use this information to adjust their strategies.

Say Yes to Political Involvement

For those involved in lobbying for pharmacists, I have respect rather than criticism. I support political action groups for pharmacists, and I am involved in advocacy and volunteer lobbying at the state level. As a teacher and advisor for a chapter of Phi Lambda Sigma (the national pharmacy leadership society), I talk with students about my lobbying days. We may discuss when you should be the 50th black suit in the room and when you should not—in other words, when to stand out so you'll be remembered and when to blend into the crowd. Or I may assign a lesson on writing and talking to the point or using only key details. Most important, I see and argue both sides of an issue. A few students comment each year that I should give my personal opinion more often, and I take that as a compliment. When teaching advocacy and lobbying to my pharmacy students, I ask them the same eye-opening question I was asked during my first interview, and I receive the same reaction that I had back then: silence and head scratching.

My first year exploring politics with students was the year the Medicare Prescription Drug Improvement and Modernization Act became law. Students were indifferent at first, but now they work side by side with me to enter patients' medications into the Centers for Medicare and Medicaid Services Web site and enroll them in the appropriate Medicare Part D plan.

Whether you choose to advocate, lobby, or financially support those who do, the key is to be involved. Don't let pharmacists become invisible. When you are not present for a group or committee meeting or do not provide input, your voice and message are not heard. Don't let this happen to pharmacists. Advocate for your profession and stay involved.

References

1. Siess JA. *The Visible Librarian: Asserting Your Value with Marketing and Advocacy.* Chicago: American Library Association; 2003.
2. Pear R. Medicare law prompts a rush for lobbyists. *The New York Times.* August 19, 2005; Section A, National Desk page 1.
3. Loomis AJ, Cigler BA. Introduction. In: Loomis AJ, Cigler BA, eds. *Interest Group Politics.* 4th ed. Washington, DC: CQ Press (division of Congressional Quarterly, Inc); 1995.
4. Seibert T. Ethics bill becomes law: aim is to control money, influence. *The Tennessean.* February 16, 2006; 102(47):1–2.
5. Levin C. Foreword. In: Luneburg WV, Susman TM, eds. *The Lobbying Manual.* 3rd ed. Chicago: American Bar Association; 2005:xxv.
6. McGrath C. Towards a lobbying profession: developing the industry's reputation, education and representation. *J Public Aff.* 2005 May;5:124–35.
7. Wolpe BC. The five commandments. In: Moore JL, ed. *Lobbying Congress: How the System Works.* Washington, DC: Congressional Quarterly, Inc; 1990.
8. Johnson DW. *Congress Online: Bridging the Gap Between Citizens and Their Representatives.* New York: Routledge; 2004.

COMMITTING TO GRASSROOTS ADVOCACY

Cynthia J. Boyle and Earlene E. Lipowski

D o you have doubts about how much influence you actually have as one person in a nation of millions? As Director of Government and Professional Affairs for the American College of Clinical Pharmacy, C. Edwin "Ed" Webb, PharmD, MPH, is a strong proponent of increasing the political advocacy capabilities and effectiveness of his organization and its members. He uses the following example to explain how influential one person can be with a member of the U.S. Congress:

> If a Congressperson represents approximately 633,000 people in a particular congressional district and the nonvoters under 18 are subtracted, 465,000 remain. Of those, 70% (325,000) are registered to vote. With 54% turnout, 175,000 actually vote. Of these, 65% (114,000) vote for the successful candidate. Fewer than 10% of these people (11,000) have donated $200 to the campaign, and of these, fewer than 10% (1,000) have donated 10 hours to the campaign. The numbers may vary by election or level of government, but these 1,000 people are much more influential than their individual votes. Grassroots advocates are influential.

Cynthia J. Boyle

Background

Cynthia J. Boyle is a faculty member at the University of Maryland School of Pharmacy and director of the School's Experiential Learning Program. She earned her Bachelor of Science degree in pharmacy from the University of Oklahoma (OU) College of Pharmacy and her PharmD from the University of Maryland. She has worked in community, institutional, and consultant pharmacy practice. As advisor for the pharmacy school's Student Government Association and through the course Effective Leadership and Advocacy, she seeks to develop leadership in 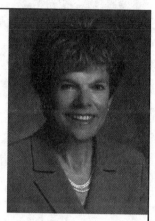 students for their future roles as advocates for patients, the profession, and public health.

Boyle was honored as the 2002 Pharmacist of the Year by the Maryland Society of Health-System Pharmacists. Long active in the Maryland Pharmacists Association (MPhA), she is the 2006–07 Chair of the Past Presidents Council. Her resolution introduced in the 2000 MPhA House of Delegates led to formation of the Maryland Pharmacy Coalition (MPC), which she chaired in 2004–05. Her leadership has been recognized through her election as 2007–08 chair of the American Pharmacists Association (APhA) Academy of Pharmacy Practice and Management Administrative Section, designation as a Fellow of APhA, selection for the 2004 LKS/Merck Vanguard Leadership Award, and service as 2005–06 president of the Phi Lambda Sigma pharmacy leadership society.

Personal Statement

I have always been active in leadership and advocacy, from high school to OU and then as a pharmacist. However, like many pharmacists after graduation, I moved away from my roots—from Oklahoma to Florida, Texas, and eventually Maryland. It takes time to develop an understanding of the political environment in a new state and to affiliate with the state pharmacy organization in a meaningful way. In retrospect, I wish I had done both sooner.

My daughter Kate had a strong influence on me when, during her final year in high school, she served as a page in the Maryland General Assembly. Her behind-the-scenes stories about legislators and the political process reignited my zeal to get involved and to help others do the same.

I have found it most advantageous to develop a solid relationship with my state delegate and to interact regularly with other elected officials throughout the year, not just during the election season. That means reviewing regular messages from my delegate on her list server, providing information to her, visiting her legislative office, contributing to her campaigns, and attending her fundraisers. One fundraiser she hosts regularly is a dessert reception held at an historic inn in Annapolis just before the start of the General Assembly session in January. Each year at that event, I meet state police officers, developers, teachers, environmentalists, and other citizens who also want to support a legislator who has been working hard and effectively on behalf of all of us and our various agendas. When I speak to the delegate, I have to be clear on whether I am speaking as an individual, a member of MPhA, or an educator.

In addition to the resources from my state and national pharmacy organizations, the MPC has helped me to keep informed about timely issues and to network for greater results than I could attain as an individual. I have learned more patience than I had before, because legislation takes time to pass, and I have tried to encourage less experienced pharmacists and student pharmacists in advocacy efforts. Although any given issue can be challenging and frustrating, grassroots advocacy is invigorating and satisfying when problems are resolved through the collegial efforts of pharmacists, student pharmacists, allies, and legislators.

Earlene E. Lipowski

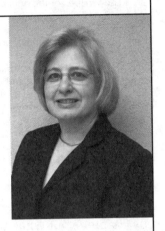

Background

Earlene Lipowski is Associate Professor of Pharmacy Health Care Administration at the University of Florida. She served as 2004–05 president of the American Pharmacists Association Academy of Pharmaceutical Research and Science. As an American Association of Colleges of Pharmacy–American Association for the Advancement of Science Congressional Fellow in 1997–98, she worked as a legislative assistant to the majority staff of the U.S. Senate Health, Education, Labor, and Pensions Committee.

Personal Statement

I've always been interested in participating in a vigorous discussion and contributing my point of view, but two events prompted my interest in political advocacy. The first was my experience as a research assistant to the Wisconsin Medicaid Evaluation Project while I was a graduate student at the University of Wisconsin (UW)–Madison. That experience taught me that there were good people doing their best to craft policy who were receptive to informative input to that process. The second event, and the turning point for me, was meeting a fellow academic (Lisa Gwyther of Duke University) who was serving 1 year as a congressional staff member in the U.S. Senate. Although there are many things one can learn from reading books, I've found that an understanding of the political process is best gained through close observation and participation.

Many people have encouraged my interest: my family, who supported my activities and cheered me on, and colleagues like Professor Bob Hammel and Joe Wiederholt and Ted Collins from my days at UW-Madison. None of these men ever walked away from an opportunity to exchange views, and for that I am grateful to all three. The best advice I ever got was the response to my asking where a person begins. The sage reply was, "It is like riding a merry-go-round: you just pick a horse, climb aboard, and start riding."

My advice to those who are interested in getting involved in advocacy is to seek to understand before seeking to be understood. A person who understands the pros and cons of an issue will be able to find win–win solutions to contentious issues. A person who understands that there is more than one way to view an issue will recognize that his or her position will not always prevail, and will not get discouraged. When you can acknowledge that well-intentioned people have legitimate but different perspectives, you develop a true appreciation for the meaning of democracy. The mistakes I have made can be traced back to my failure to truly listen to my opponent's point of view.

For me, advocacy is not an activity that is added on to my professional responsibilities; rather, it is a part of my professional responsibility. Therefore, I do not have to carve out additional time for advocacy. I advise pharmacy students to do three things to be an effective advocate. First, read every issue (monthly or weekly) of one professional publication from cover to cover; skim other professional publications and read selected articles of interest. Second, read a good newspaper, or the online equivalent, daily. Third, follow one issue—just one. Choosing a single issue makes the goal manageable. Furthermore, it is not hard to find one issue of particular interest to you or your practice, and in the process of following its development, you will come to better understand the policy and advocacy process.

All the professional pharmacy associations have legislative staff members who can provide background and up-to-date information about matters of interest. I rely on all of them; some groups have a broad perspective on the issues, while others focus more narrowly on topics of concern to specific practice types or settings. In my opinion, the very best resource for following health policy issues outside pharmacy is the Kaiser Family Foundation, which offers tutorials, comprehensive reports, surveys, data, and current events through a variety of Web sites all accessible at www.kff.org, including a section devoted specifically to prescription drugs.

The term "grassroots advocacy" has appeared in several previous chapters, but what does it really mean in relation to political activism? Simply stated, the grassroots are the local areas where advocates live and vote or where their organization or group conducts business. Think about how grass grows and how it spreads, and you will see how the term grassroots advocacy emerged.

Effective grassroots advocates look for fertile ground and the best possible environment in which to advocate. They spread enthusiasm to others, just as grass sends out runners. They may venture where people are not familiar with their points of view (sparse areas) and rejoice when their ideas take root. Even experienced grassroots advocates need regular interaction with other advocates to maintain focus and to stay current on the issues. Many times, advocacy efforts do not go as planned, and issues go dormant. In such a case, dedicated and persistent advocates monitor the legislative and regulatory environments for opportunities to revitalize their cause.

Getting Started in Grassroots Advocacy

Now that you understand that your voice will be heard, let us look at how it can be effective. If you want to have an impact on issues at any level—local, state, or national—you can do this through grassroots advocacy, a term many people have used interchangeably with volunteer lobbying. As explained in Chapter 10, lobbying, whether volunteer or paid, is a type of grassroots advocacy but more directly involves influencing the introduction of legislation and voting behavior. As a grassroots advocate, you may act as a citizen, a member of a community group, an employee or executive in a business, a member of a trade or professional group, a member of a public interest group, or a participant in a private-sector interest group.

"I have an issue."   Advocacy is needed at several points in the legislative process. At the outset, it is important to establish awareness of the issue. It is difficult to predict when and why a given issue will spark the interest of legislators or citizens. Interest can arise through a shared personal experience with relatives and friends. A media story often sparks citizens' inquiries and draws matters to the attention of legislators. This stage of advocacy can be frustrating, because it is easy to become discouraged in the face of apparent indifference or an inadequate response to a particular issue. However, specific incidents, such as medication errors reported on the evening news, capture the public's attention and may generate a call to action precisely because of a nagging concern, a sense of outrage, or even fear. Once an issue has been identified, coordinated actions with others of like mind and persistence become important.

"I have a proposal."   When the moment is right, you must be prepared to take action. Public attention is fleeting, and the only safe prediction is that others will be ready to take action when you least expect it or when you are preoccupied with other matters. This is the Murphy's Law of politics! When the legislator or public official surprises you with an expression of support for action, you must be prepared with a response. Persons who have thought and communicated about an issue are in a better position to advance a promising remedy. Action is more likely to follow if a written proposal can be placed on the table and negotiations begun while the interest is at its peak. Drafting a proposal in the proper format of a bill is not a brash step; quite the opposite is true. Having a concrete proposal waiting in the portfolio demonstrates that an advocate is sincere and has given matters considerable thought before entering the political arena. The bill will most likely be rewritten along the way, but it is always best to establish a starting point for discussion of feasibility.

"I have considered financial impact."   Being prepared to suggest a legislative solution requires consideration of the fiscal impact. Legislation may change policy without financial ramifications, or it may include new programs with financial consequences. A common mistake is not understanding the difference. For example, a bill to designate pharmacists as providers is not simply a change in a state's practice act; it has financial implications for credentialing pharmacists and monitoring their activities.

At the federal level, no bill can be put up for a vote without being assessed by the Congressional Budget Office. Bills introduced after the adoption of the annual budget resolution must be cost neutral. That is, while budgets are being drafted, funding requests are generally on equal footing. Once the body has parceled out sums of money for specific sectors such as education, transportation, security, and health, new proposals will be a tradeoff with activities already endorsed. Just as a typical household budget must be reconfigured to accommodate unexpected events, a successful legislative proposal must be a substitute for or generate savings from another part of the spending plan.

Advocates are best prepared if they can propose steps that do not require substantial expenditures. Such suggestions will find an eager audience, and legislators and their staff members will be pleasantly surprised. The adage is that every problem could be fixed if only we could spend more money. Well-intentioned public servants expend enormous energy in search of low-cost solutions to common problems. They are just as frustrated as the rest of us when reminded that resources are finite.

"I have considered the legislator's point of view."   The mark of a successful elected official is consistency with his or her political platform. Since it is not possible to debate every issue in detail with the majority of voters, politicians strive for a level of consistency in their actions, and they usually have one or two areas of focus. For example, one legislator may declare a position of fiscal conservatism. The financial implications of any proposal are going to be an issue for her. Another politician may hold civil and human rights in high regard; the most likely position on any issue before him will turn on issues of civil liberty. You should know the background of your legislative contacts and be prepared to respond when they inevitably raise questions.

"I know the rules and the players."   As in a game of chess, you must be familiar with the moves that are allowed and not allowed, in addition to anticipating the moves of your opponents. Above all, your strategy must be flexible, and you must be prepared for the unexpected. You may need to line up other advocates for a campaign of last-minute phone calls to a committee, or to ask other legislators to intervene with a parliamentary procedure or other legislative tactics. Although it seems to take forever for the public to recognize the merits of your position, action can be taken at a staggering pace. Advocates may need to maintain constant contact with the legislative office or committee staff to make sure they are aware of rapid developments. A planning horizon of 1 week can be considered long-range planning when a bill is moving through the legislative process. Planning a month in advance may be wishful thinking, especially at the end of a legislative session when votes happen frequently.

Communicating with Legislators

The best advice on communicating with legislators is to present the facts and to debate with solid logic. Be honest, helpful, and accurate when talking with legislators, officials, and staff members. Treat them as intelligent individuals who want to do the right thing. Your job is to inform them what you think is right. However, debate becomes painful when the position is selfish and the arguments are self-serving. It is obvious when an individual's position is based entirely on self-interest and not on the best interests of the public.

Critical thinking skills are an asset in debating the opposition, and attention must be devoted to what is not said or explained in full. Even though political arguments are generally not regarded as precise and accurate assertions, the professional must examine the underlying assumptions, deductions, and inferences that are drawn. Point out the flaws in your opponent's position. Opponents in a fair fight will not fault you for promoting your cause and stating your position forcefully.

Those who have been fortunate enough to obtain legislative action on a matter of interest should by no means reduce their efforts and attention to their cause. All complex problems and human endeavors are fraught with challenges. Much can go awry during the regulation phase (discussed in a previous chapter) and program implementation. In the rare instance in which a new policy or law is implemented with few problems, inevitable changes in technology, the economy, and social trends will require grassroots advocates to revisit the issue. In fact, you may find that nearly all of your advocacy efforts and communication can focus on the untoward effects of well-intentioned legislation that has generated them, rather than on entirely new initiatives.

Some people are cynical and express anger, frustration, and disgust with the notion of lobbying or grassroots advocacy. But an effective grassroots advocate is positive and constructive, offering logical solutions to complex problems. An advocate with a healthy attitude focuses on the process and gets involved because information about preferences and needs must be transmitted from citizens to the government officials who make policy decisions. For our democratic system to work, expressing our views to someone in a position to take legislative action is necessary; and in our representative form of government, legislators cannot represent you without your input. It is your responsibility, especially as a professional, to respond to an issue on which you have specialized knowledge or expertise.

Expressing Your Position in Person: Where and How

Individual legislators are most familiar with three types of bills: (1) those they personally sponsor, (2) those that come before committees on which they serve, and (3) those that someone in their district has urged them to either support or oppose. Remember that, as a constituent, you are in the unique position of being able to express the views of the district to the legislator, so local stories and angles are particularly useful. Communicating with elected representatives by inviting them to visit a pharmacy work setting to see pharmaceutical care in action is highly recommended. Elected officials listen closely, particularly when they are on home turf and have allocated time to getting in touch with the people they represent.

Members of Congress and state legislatures generally leave the capital on Friday afternoon to return to their home state or district. Most elected representatives know that it is critical to stay in touch with the mood and thinking of the constituents back home. Local officials, too, must set aside time to mingle with their constituents. Those who do not interact with their constituents are not likely to be in office in the next election cycle. Members of the public should take advantage of these opportunities to express their opinions and share their knowledge. Later, when mulling over policy options, elected representatives will be able to relate them to real life experiences.

Individual appointments.   If there is no designated forum available for communicating with an elected official, you can make an appointment to meet with the official. Start any meeting by establishing rapport. For example, you might thank the legislator for a past vote or for the opportunity to meet. Provide your business card.

Group appointments.   Decide ahead of time which member of the group will make a brief presentation on your topic. Always have the facts straight and use them to support your position. Use a one-page fact sheet, letter, or brief outline to convey your main points succinctly, and provide the name of a contact who can supply more information at a later date.

Position statements.   Make your position clear, and then ask for your legislator's position. Do not expect a commitment on the spot. Most legislators are thoughtful and deliberate. They make a practice of seeking multiple perspectives on a particular issue before taking a position. You need not settle for evasive answers, but always remain polite.

Support. If your representative immediately expresses agreement with your position, ask her or him to take leadership in convincing other less supportive members of your state's delegation. Your representative can help persuade the political leadership and other colleagues to support your position. Express appreciation for any action the representative takes on your behalf.

Disagreement.   Also accept the fact that people have honest differences of opinion. People of goodwill have different priorities. This is certainly true in the realm of health policy, since personal, ethical, cultural, emotional, social, and economic considerations are inherent in establishing a position on the issues. Always leave the door open for further discussion. Be appreciative. Legislators are inundated with requests for their time and action. It is always appropriate to thank them for listening. Remember that compromise is usually the result of controversial legislation and regulations.

Staff contacts.   At times you will not be able to see an elected official but will be offered an opportunity to meet with a member of the staff. More than 10,000 bills and resolutions are introduced in each session of Congress. Since a representative's time must be spread over the entire range of issues facing the nation, it is actually in your best interest to know the name, e-mail address, and telephone number of the staff member responsible for following health-related issues. On every Congressman's staff is a health legislative assistant who would be pleased to get to know constituents who are respected members of the community; these staff members are knowledgeable and responsive to questions.

Take an active role in educating staffers by providing information or analysis. Make yourself the trusted resource when time is short and decisions are pressing. Staff members need to see pharmacist constituents as the people to seek for explanations and for ideas to improve policy. Staff members will inform your representative about the technical aspects of policy decisions and will keep the viewpoints of various constituencies in mind when policy options are under consideration.

Although there are a few seasoned veterans in staff positions, most staff members are young, highly intelligent, well-educated, ambitious, hard working, and poorly paid employees who seek the extraordinary experiences that come with being part of the policy-making process. They often work under tremendous time pressure with scarce resources. Your input will be considered if it is accessible. If not, policy will be devised and debated and decisions made without your input.

Follow-up. Send thank-you letters as soon as possible to the representative and to the staff members who arranged or were present at your meeting. Include a brief summary of your position and answers to any questions you could not answer during the meeting, and reiterate any commitments made to you by the staff or legislator during the meeting. Be responsive if a legislator or staff person asks for more information, and provide it in a timely manner. A good relationship with a legislator and the staff will help you when you want information later. A cautionary note is warranted here. Do not present a gift to the legislator or staff during your meeting, and do not present a political action committee (PAC) contribution while discussing an issue. Both actions give the appearance of impropriety, even if the two events are unrelated.

Expressing Your Position by Phone or in Writing

Listings for offices of local, state, and federal representatives can be found in your telephone book and on the Internet. To telephone the Washington office of all Senators and Representatives, you can call the Capitol switchboard at 202-224-3121 (Senate) or 202-225-3121 (House). Know the name and number of the bill of interest. When you reach the office, ask to speak to the person dealing with the issue about which you are calling. Remember the name of the person to whom you speak; you may want to reach him or her again. This contact can give you excellent information and will report your concerns to the legislator.

Describe your issue or viewpoint in your own words, and ask what your legislator plans to do about the bill. For example, if you are calling to urge co-sponsorship, ask if the legislator will be a co-sponsor or when that decision will be made. If you cannot

Advice from a National Legislator

Senator Joseph Lieberman's book *In Praise of Public Life* provides some advice on grassroots participation in the political process. Senator Lieberman says he learned that in politics one should always strive to convince previous opponents to become supporters in the next election. The same could be said about pieces of legislation.

Senator Lieberman's approach to decisions about personal behavior and political actions is to ask not only, Is it legal? but also, Is it right? He believes every American can and should use his or her citizenship to make our government better—to make it, in the words of former President Jimmy Carter, as good as the American people are.

Senator Lieberman says citizens can elevate public life by

- Registering to vote and voting,
- Contacting elected officials and stating desires and beliefs on particular issues,
- Getting involved in campaigns for supportive candidates,
- Personally applying beliefs through some form of public or civil service, and
- Running for public office if they so desire. (Senator Lieberman's book is an excellent resource for people considering public office.)

Thoughts of a State Pharmacist-Legislator

We asked pharmacy owner Robert "Bob" Osterhaus to comment for this chapter on his experience as a legislator. Osterhaus was awarded the Remington Honor Medal, pharmacy's highest honor, for his proven leadership and his vision in promoting collaboration among the Iowa Pharmacy Association and the state's two colleges of pharmacy to form the Iowa Center for Pharmaceutical Care. His comments and advice follow:

> I became a legislator because my Republican predecessor died in the middle of his term. He had been diagnosed with cancer and successfully treated, and he intended to return to the Iowa House of Representatives in January 1996. He had been a patient at our pharmacy, and I knew him well, although we had political differences. After his death, I was asked by the Democratic Party to run for the unexpired term in a special election. I agreed to run December 27, and by January 18 I was seated as a state representative in Des Moines. The unexpired term would end that November, and since I had planned to serve no more than 3 years, I next ran for office for the 2-year term. My most highly contested election was the first one; I had token

opposition the other four times I ran. I wound up staying 9 years, all of which were spent in the minority party. Because of my community involvement in my rural area and my name recognition, I was lucky to never experience a close election. During all 9 years, I was the only pharmacist in the Iowa legislature, and now there is none.

My approach to elected state office was to not act like a politician. I did my sinning in public, meaning that if I had a drink with someone, it would be at a local bar. I never felt like I had to have the job, and that gave me flexibility. I listened to the people, provided service, and took positions and expressed them. People may not agree, but they respect a politician who honestly explains his or her stance.

I had no desire for higher office. I have noticed that, like coaches and celebrities, legislators sometimes stay too long in office. For politicians, especially senators, there is so much power and prestige in office that it can be hard to step down and return to private life.

It does take money to run for office. The Iowa Democratic Party helped me in my first election but expected to be reimbursed. I had worked with the American Pharmacists Association (APhA) PAC board, and APhA helped publicize my candidacy. Pharmacists from across the country contributed to my Iowa campaigns.

My success as a pharmacist-legislator came because of timing, a willingness to consider elected office and change plans, and, especially, a supportive wife. Ann stood by my decisions and in fact acted as my clerk in the legislature. In Iowa, legislators do not have offices. We have a desk and a two-drawer filing cabinet in the chamber. The legislative session runs 3 to 4 months, until April. Some legislators have as much as a 4½ hour commute to the capital, but we were able to go home on weekends. Most weeks I would be in Des Moines Monday through Thursday and would attend forums or events over the weekend. Even after the legislative session, a legislator must research issues, resolve questions, conduct committee business, and provide constituent services. I also enjoyed reading about other states' issues and meeting legislators at national meetings.

I had to be more than a pharmacist. My legislative focus was health care issues, on which I had a unique perspective, especially on Medicaid and mental health. For 8 years, I was the ranking member of the appropriations subcommittee for human services, but I could not be an expert in only that area. I also had to become knowledgeable about transportation, insurance, agriculture, schools, and the environment. I learned to defend my positions, and I enjoyed discussions, particularly those related to children's health. I am proudest of the Iowa Hawk-I child health plan.

One thing is frequently overlooked in grassroots efforts. Experienced legislators will ask grassroots advocates, "Who is opposed to this?" You must be ready to respond. In my case the opponent would often be the insurance industry. I gave up trying to work with them! My best advice is to know who you are and why you believe what you do.

reach the appropriate staff member, leave a clear message with the receptionist, explaining that you are a constituent and that you want the representative to take specific action on a particular bill.

When writing to your legislator, use the same strategy. Use your own words and stationery. Include your home address and sign your name legibly. Try to keep your letter to one page. Do not worry about receiving a form letter in response. Popular issues that generate a lot of correspondence often are handled by interns and volunteers. A letter from a health care professional that addresses an issue in detail will be routed to a legislative assistant. In either case, you can rest assured that your opinion has been noted.

Communication from constituents, whether by mail or phone, is typically reported in weekly logs that keep representatives updated on the amount of correspondence arriving on each side of current issues. These logs are indicators of the atmosphere in their districts, and just a few letters on one bill can make a legislator pay attention to it.

Association Strategies for Grassroots Advocacy

Even within a single profession such as pharmacy, myriad issues exist among personal and professional interests. As association members, pharmacists and student pharmacists can shape advocacy positions by responding to opinion polls and surveys, as well as participating in committee work at the state or national level. Many organizations have a PAC, as mentioned in Chapter 8. Most PACs provide modest contributions to political candidates whose positions are supportive, but PACs serve more broadly through efforts to educate members about the issues and the procedures through which laws and regulations are created.

Many of us are not eager to take on the challenge of advocacy or volunteer lobbying, but there is plenty of support to make the task less daunting. National professional associations strive to keep members current on issues and provide relevant background information. They employ a professional policy and advocacy staff dedicated to working on our behalf. They maintain contact with key congressional staff and know the policy positions of elected officials. In state organizations, the association executive director may play a similar role, staying in touch with key legislators and tracking specific pieces of legislation. Keeping informed can be as simple as joining a political information network. A network usually will send a monthly legislative and regulatory newsletter supplemented with occasional announcements about new developments. Effective associations develop an advocacy

As a grassroots advocate, you may act as a citizen, a member of a community group, an employee or executive in a business, a member of a trade or professional group, a member of a public interest group, or a participant in a private-sector interest group.

and outreach communication strategy in advance, especially for fast-breaking matters. Strategic alliances with other pharmacists and advocates generate synergistic effects, as long as the communication network does not break down when some people are unavailable or engaged in other issues.

Nonprofit organizations, including many pharmacy organizations, are prohibited from direct lobbying under the Internal Revenue Service (IRS) regulations that define nonprofit status and distinguish between direct and grassroots lobbying. Tax laws establish what an organization and its officers may and may not do when acting on behalf of the organization. It is beyond the scope of this text to go into depth on this issue, but association members and officers should become familiar with the Exempt Organizations Tax Manual (Chapter 27 at www.irs.gov) and seek the advice of counsel in order to ensure compliance with tax laws, including appropriate accounting procedures for reporting allocations of dues and other income.

Commitment:
10 Steps toward Active Advocacy

Most pharmacists are able to find more than enough activities to fill their work life. It is difficult to imagine how we can find the time and energy to make room for advocacy. Perhaps the best approach is not to add more activities but to cultivate an appreciation of how our current activities are forms of advocacy. As with any journey, the most difficult step is the first one. Here are some examples of how you can embark on the road from passive to more active advocacy.

1. Follow *one* policy issue related to pharmacy that attracts your interest—just one. Make an effort to read each news article and editorial you encounter on the subject; attend a presentation on the topic or watch a special feature on television. (The secret is that virtually all of the issues you could select are interrelated. You will learn about a wide scope of policy issues just by following the one you choose.)
2. Read *one* pharmacy journal every month cover to cover—your choice! Skim the table of contents in other publications and then read only those items of special interest.
3. When you encounter a person who needs an advocate, take *one* action on his or her behalf. This person could be a patient, a student pharmacist, or a colleague.
4. Vote in an election. That is, fill out and submit a ballot for something such as electing officers for a professional organization, changing the bylaws of your neighborhood association, or electing the next President of the United States.
5. Participate in professional committees when your help is requested; attend meetings regularly to voice your thoughts and opinions on important matters that affect your practice.
6. Form *one* strategic alliance with an individual or a group as a way to advance your personal self-interest. For example, negotiate or collaborate toward a win–win resolution to a problem with your co-worker.
7. Set down goals for personal professional development, including one activity that will enhance your leadership skills, and assess your progress at least annually.

8. Write *one* letter to the editor of a journal, editor of a newspaper, local or state official, state legislator, member of Congress, or business manager. This need not be a complaint; letters of congratulation and expressions of appreciation count.
9. Run for an office (APhA-Academy of Student Pharmacists, student government association, county council, state delegate).
10. Visit the legislative section of one pharmacy organization's Web site, or subscribe to an e-mail legislative report from a pharmacy organization.

Conclusion

Advocacy and outreach must be ongoing efforts, building long-term relationships. Persistent grassroots advocacy will gain recognition of pharmacists as health care providers who can solve medication-use problems. Effective grassroots advocates in pharmacy will not only reinforce to citizens that pharmacists are concerned with improving the health of the public, but will also demonstrate the political impact of the profession. Pharmacists advocate for patients, but patients are also some of the best advocates for pharmacy. Grassroots advocates build connections, networks, and even friendships as they work toward the results they seek.

Additional Resources

American Association of Colleges of Pharmacy Joint Committee on Advocacy and Outreach. Sagraves R, Lipowski E, co-chairs. Final Report. July 2005.

Avner M. *The Lobbying and Advocacy Handbook for Nonprofit Organizations*. St. Paul, Minn: Wilder Foundation; 2002.

Boyle CJ. Developing the grassroots advocate. *J Am Pharm Assoc.* 2004;44:5–6.

Lipowski EE. Lobbying can lead to acknowledgment as health care providers. *J Am Pharm Assoc.* 2004;44:6.

BRIDGING STATE AND FEDERAL ADVOCACY

Arnold E. Clayman and Joseph Hill

M ost of the rules and regulations that affect pharmacist practitioners on a daily basis have their origin in national issues that find their way down to the state level. The source may be federal legislation or regulations that must be adopted by the states, or national movements on issues that begin in one particular state. Bridging the gap from national issues to state implementation requires advocacy by pharmacists in their respective states. Without involvement at the grassroots level, pharmacists may find themselves dealing with rules and regulations that are difficult to implement in their daily practice. Helping to shape workable rules of practice through advocacy by practitioners from different areas of pharmacy can be a most satisfying and rewarding experience.

Differences between Federal and State Lawmaking

In many respects, statehouses across the country are smaller versions of Congress. Most states have bicameral legislatures (two separate bodies, such as a house and senate); Nebraska is the lone

Arnold E. Clayman

Background

After receiving his bachelor of science degree from the University of Maryland School of Pharmacy, Arnold "Arnie" Clayman spent 11 years on the staff of the University of Maryland Medical Center Hospital. In 1984 he opened the Mid-Atlantic branch of a home infusion company. Since 1988, he has been involved in long-term care (LTC), continuing to develop infusion as a part of comprehensive pharmacy services to patients and residents both in facilities and at home.

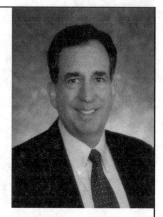

An American Society of Consultant Pharmacists (ASCP) member since 1988, Clayman is a current member of the ASCP Board of Directors, Board liaison to the Government Affairs Committee, and a member of the National Association of Boards of Pharmacy/Drug Enforcement Administration task force. He reorganized the Maryland ASCP chapter (MD-ASCP), served as its president for 3 years, and now serves on its board of directors. He chairs the chapter's legislative committee and, with the Maryland Pharmacy Coalition, plans the legislative day every year in Annapolis. In 2000 he was recognized by MD-ASCP with the Pharmacist of the Year Award and in November 2004 was awarded the ASCP Richard S. Berman Service Award. He currently serves as a preceptor for the geriatric pharmacy practice residency jointly sponsored by the University of Maryland and MD-ASCP.

Personal Statement

It's interesting how our road in life takes us places we may never have imagined going. I was politically conscious of the issues of the late 1960s and the 1970s, but I wasn't aware of the regulatory issues the pharmacy profession faced. In 1988 I attended my first national meeting of ASCP and suddenly discovered that pharmacists can have passion about their profession. ASCP Executive Director Tim Webster inspired me to get involved and really care about the future of our profession. He was a visionary who saw what might be and tried to make it happen.

I was introduced to advocacy while I was MD-ASCP president and thus the official representative of LTC pharmacy in Maryland. I was asked to participate in committees, task forces, and any forum where LTC pharmacy needed a voice. It was a humbling experience and put me in situations beyond my comfort level, especially when it came to legislative and political issues. Until then, I had no great interest in these areas, but over time I grew to understand the importance of being involved in the process and how it can change the way we practice on a daily basis. Unless we are involved, others will be making decisions for us—something that pharmacists are always complaining about.

My leadership skills were developed in the area of performing arts before I applied them to pharmacy professional organizations. I had produced plays for a theater group and concerts for a music group, and I had learned to manage hundreds of volunteers and staff to put on a performance that aspired to be both artistically and financially successful. I used this approach in forming committees on various topics. When an organization starts to become very proficient, it becomes easy for members to keep doing a job and not involve others in committee work. Then, when these leaders start to lose interest, an organization without strong committees must suddenly start looking for new blood to keep going. I have seen this mistake happen many times. Another important leadership skill is consensus building; you have very little control over volunteers other than their interest. There is a fine line between letting people express their points of view and making decisions for an organization; if either of these is taken to an extreme, the organization won't work.

Recognizing my efforts at the state level, ASCP leaders encouraged me to get more involved at the national level. Again, this wasn't something to which I had aspired. I have advocated for pharmacy on the state and national levels and have felt grateful for the opportunity to make a difference. A high school teacher once told me that the journey of a thousand miles begins with the first step. Now I truly understand what that means.

Joseph Hill

Background

Joseph Hill represents the American Society of Consultant Pharmacists (ASCP) before state and federal legislators and regulators. He serves as spokesman for ASCP's policy priorities for senior care pharmacy. Before joining ASCP, he was Director of State Legislative Affairs for the American Association of Health Plans and Associate Director of State Legislative Affairs for the Healthcare Distribution Management Association.

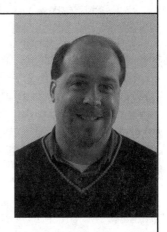

Personal Statement

When I was growing up, my father was an attorney who served as legal counsel to the Pennsylvania State Senate Transportation Committee. After hearing his stories and witnessing his excitement about the process, I became more and more interested in politics and government.

I studied political science at both the undergraduate and graduate levels. I was able to serve as an intern for a Pennsylvania senator in Harrisburg and got a firsthand look at policy making. In my professional life, I have had the experience of working on state and federal issues, as well as on grassroots and political fundraising. It is extremely rewarding to be a part of the political process and work toward solutions that improve the practice of pharmacy and, ultimately, the lives of the patients pharmacists serve.

One of the most effective techniques I have found is having a network of interested parties that can share information and work together on issues. Politics and government are based on relationships and social interaction. Having a wide network of friends and contacts helps ensure open communication and information sharing.

One of the biggest mistakes I've made was very early in my career. I was working on an issue in Delaware, but I was not following the lead of our contacts on the ground in Dover. I have since learned that the "We're from Washington and we're here to fix what isn't broken" approach does not bode well for establishing and maintaining strong state relationships.

> *Bridging the gap from national issues to state implementation requires advocacy by pharmacists in their respective states. Without involvement at the grassroots level, pharmacists may find themselves dealing with rules and regulations that are difficult to implement in their daily practice.*

exception. All of these legislative bodies perform the same function—passing laws—although there are differences between federal and state legislative activity.

The agenda in Congress is national in scope, focusing on problems occurring across the country. Many of these are the high-profile issues, such as foreign conflicts, spikes in gasoline prices, and economic pressures involving unemployment or inflation. Furthermore, the influence of the media is greater at the federal level. In addition, there are many times when Congress must respond to issues that emerge outside its regular schedule.

Legislative agendas at the state level are largely driven by budget cycles. Except in Vermont, every state legislature is required by law to pass a budget before adjourning for the year. This places tremendous pressure on the legislators. As a result, late in the session states tend to shift focus to the budget while other issues fall by the wayside. This means that your particular issue must be introduced as early as possible and should be moving through the process prior to budget negotiations. At the same time, if your livelihood depends upon state funding (providing health care under Medicaid, for example), you must be vigilant during those last few weeks of budget talks to be sure that cuts will not affect your reimbursement. Last-minute cuts happen quickly and usually are not widely publicized. Eleventh-hour deal making is common, because legislators are in a rush to adjourn for the year.

Unlike the federal government, most states still have part-time legislatures, and a few of them (Texas, Arkansas, Montana, Nevada, Oregon, and North Dakota) meet only every other year. There are just nine full-time state legislatures, so most state lawmakers have jobs outside their public service.

The bridge between federal and state-level activity can be manifested in two basic ways, examples of which are provided below. The first is when regulations or legislation enacted federally must be implemented by each state. This normally happens rapidly, since most regulations have specific implementation dates. The second is when ideas or programs enacted by a state gain popularity and spread to other states. Implementation may spread rapidly or may take years to reach a majority of states. While there is only one federal government, there are 50 states—which may share the same concerns or may perceive things differently. Discussions of a given issue may vary greatly from state to state. In the past, large states such as New York and California were viewed as bellwether states; that is, when they acted, other states would follow suit. This is less true today, as smaller states are taking the lead on important issues. Still, legislators often consult their counterparts in other states for information and advice on dealing with issues in their own state.

A third type of link between national and state actions is a combination of the first two. Federal law mandates that states enact certain standards; however, states may go a step further and adopt stricter regulations than those prescribed in federal law. This approach appears to be gaining popularity throughout the country. An example is stricter state regulation of the sale of products used in the illicit manufacture of amphetamines.

Federal Actions with State-Level Implementation

National standards that may be enforced at the discretion of the Food and Drug Administration (FDA), regulations issued by the Drug Enforcement Administration (DEA), and federally granted waivers to state Medicaid programs are examples of federal actions implemented by the states. States have the power to adopt regulations from the federal agencies verbatim or to draft more stringent regulations.

Sterile compounding standards. New national standards dealing with sterile compounding, *United States Pharmacopoeia* (USP) Chapter 797: Pharmaceutical Compounding—Sterile Preparations, became effective in 2004. The intent was to present the first enforceable standards for sterile compounding in all practice settings; the chapter was developed after many years of drafting recommendations and professional guidelines to enhance patient safety. The chapter addresses the physical environment as well as procedural requirements for the safe compounding of sterile products. While USP is a standards-setting organization, the standards themselves can be enforced by FDA. Early on, FDA said it would not directly enforce pharmacies' compliance with any of the USP chapters on compounding. Rather, FDA exercises what it calls enforcement discretion, preferring to confront pharmacies whose preparation of items meets the agency's definition of manufacturing. FDA does not license or inspect pharmacies on a state level, so it is up to each individual state board of pharmacy to develop regulations that satisfy the USP standards.

Some states have taken the approach of simply referencing the USP standards in their regulations. This approach places an additional burden on pharmacy license holders and state inspectors to learn and apply the USP standards.

Other states have taken a different approach by developing their own regulations based on the USP Chapter 797 standards. The Maryland Board of Pharmacy, for example, developed its own version of the USP standards. In January 2005 the board convened a sterile compounding task force to develop the regulations, with representatives from the various pharmacy practice settings (hospital, long-term care, and community practice) that prepare sterile compounds. The task force gathered similar regulations from other states that had gone through this process. It developed regulations, as well as tools for state pharmacy inspectors, to be enacted by the board of pharmacy.

Controlled-substance prescribing in long-term care. Another example involves regulatory changes made by DEA concerning controlled prescriptions for residents of long-term care facilities (LTCFs). In an emergency, a prescription for a Schedule II medication can be telephoned to the pharmacist in a community pharmacy, as long as this is followed with a written copy signed by the prescriber within

72 hours. For patients in LTCFs, the time was extended from 72 hours to 7 days, and faxed orders signed by the prescriber could be accepted as originals. The federal regulations have now been changed again—from 72 hours to 7 days for all pharmacy practice settings—but the fax exception for LTCFs is still in effect. Even though these were federal changes in regulation, each state had to enact the change into its controlled-drug regulations.

Medicaid waivers.   As Medicaid is set up, federal law sets forth the basic structure of the program, along with an agreement to assist states with funding of the program. States, in turn, govern the day-to-day operations of the program, such as determining coverage restrictions and reimbursement levels to providers. However, states may make more substantive changes to their Medicaid programs by obtaining permission from the federal government (that is, requesting a waiver). States petition the federal agency that governs Medicaid, the Centers for Medicare and Medicaid Services (CMS), to make changes in their Medicaid programs. If the waivers are approved, the changes can be made. These tend to be changes in the structure of the program, such as enabling a state to impose some limited cost sharing on certain beneficiaries or allowing private managed care insurance plans to provide coverage and cost containment.

This state–federal partnership presents enormous challenges for those who provide health care services under Medicaid. Not only must you, as a provider, be aware of the requirements of your state (and any other state in which you practice), but you must be aware of how the program is governed at the federal level as well. Many health care provider trade associations and professional societies have staff devoted solely to tracking federal and state changes in Medicaid. Imagine having a practice that operates in all 50 states: You would theoretically have to track all 50 states and the federal government to keep abreast of changes in the program.

State Programs that Spread Nationwide

Pharmacists' authority to immunize patients and to engage in collaborative drug therapy management are examples of legislative gains in one state that spread to others.

Immunization by pharmacists.   Over the past 30 years many professional health care associations, advocacy groups, and government health agencies in the United States have worked to improve the public's access to immunizations. One method of expanding access is allowing pharmacists to administer vaccines. Since administering injections is outside the pharmacist's traditional scope of practice, states needed to change their regulations to allow pharmacists to immunize patients. This initiative has spread across the country state by state, aided by the advocacy of local pharmacists. Local efforts have been supported by programs of the national professional associations, such as the 100% Immunization Campaign coordinated by the American Society of Consultant Pharmacists (ASCP) and the Pharmacy-Based Immunization Certificate Program of the American Pharmacists Association (APhA). The specifics of practice differ from state to state, but more than 40 states have made changes in their pharmacy practice acts to allow pharmacists to administer immunizations.

Collaborative drug therapy management.   Because of the growing awareness that pharmacists' specialized knowledge and abilities contribute to quality patient care, collaborative practice or collaborative drug therapy management (CDTM) agreements are being used in many states. CDTM involves a voluntary written agreement between a pharmacist and one or more prescribers that permits an expanded scope of practice for the pharmacist, such as the ability to initiate or modify drug therapy and order laboratory tests. These agreements usually include protocols, practice guidelines, care plans, and formulary systems, which in some cases need to be approved by state agencies before they can be put into practice.

Starting with pilot projects in the 1970s, CDTM began to catch people's attention; by 1977 California had passed legislation to allow this practice for pharmacists involved in a specific project. This was expanded in 1981 when California allowed a larger group of pharmacists to participate in specific CDTM activities. The state of Washington authorized pharmacist participation in CDTM under protocol in 1979. In 1986 the Florida legislature created a third class of drugs for pharmacists to use in treating patients with acute illnesses. Today over 40 states have some sort of CDTM in their regulations.

Developing legislation and regulations to allow these collaborative agreements to exist has been a challenge in some states. Hard-fought efforts have involved pharmacists from many practice settings. The national pharmacy associations and practitioners from other states have helped by testifying before subcommittees of the legislatures considering these bills. In some cases, the physician and nursing communities have been opposed to this expansion of the pharmacist's scope of practice, and the bills have been defeated. Pharmacy groups have learned from their mistakes and made additional attempts.

In Maryland, the term "collaborative practice" elicited such fierce opposition that it was changed to "drug therapy management," and physicians and nurses were invited to participate in a task force assembled to draft specific language within the bill. Using a more conservative scope of allowable practices and requiring more oversight from both pharmacy and medical boards, along with strong advocacy efforts, enabled the bill to be passed by the state senate. As the bill moved to the house of delegates, it received some vocal opposition from physicians and was sent to a task force for resolution of certain issues, but eventually, during the 2002 session, it was passed by both houses of the Maryland legislature. Maryland pharmacists worked for more than 10 years to bring this national trend to fruition in their state.

Stricter Regulation by States

During the 1990s, methamphetamine users were manufacturing the drug by purchasing nonprescription (over-the-counter) cough and cold products and using their active ingredients to make methamphetamine in home labs. In response, states sought to limit access to these cough and cold products by either placing them behind the counter or requiring a prescription to obtain them. The states shared information on what worked to make these products less accessible to those who would abuse them. This issue began, however, with the enactment of a federal law called the Methamphetamine Control Act of 1995 ("Combat Meth Act"). That law established basic requirements for the sale of nonprescription cough and cold products used to make methamphetamine. States were required to have minimum restrictions in place, but they were free to enact more restrictive laws than the federal law.

The result was that states began enacting laws that imposed lower quantity limits on the sale of these products than were required under federal law. The idea was to further restrict the quantity that a person could purchase at any one time. In addition, states worked across borders to gather information and discuss ways to stem methamphetamine production. Oregon went so far as to require a prescription for purchase of these products. Not to be outdone, in 2006 Congress rolled the provisions of the Combat Meth Act into the reauthorization of the USA Patriot Act. There are now federal standards that limit the amount of cough and cold products containing pseudoephedrine that can be purchased by an individual at retail.

Strength in Numbers

Benjamin Franklin once said, "We must, indeed, all hang together or, most assuredly, we shall all hang separately." This statement is as true today as it was during the American Revolution. Advocacy, whether at the state or federal level, is generally more effective when the entire group of stakeholders, not just one or two persons, can be activated. This is done by garnering resources and mobilizing those who share similar concerns about an issue. To begin, ask yourself these questions: What is the issue (bill or regulation) and its impact? Who is affected by it? Where is it in the process? Finally, why is it an issue, or what has occurred to make it a perceived problem? This approach can help you identify critical issues, recognize those who share your concerns, provide background on the issue, and find cooperative strategies for resolving the problem.

A major function of health care trade associations and professional societies is bringing together stakeholders and providing forums where they can share experiences and explore solutions. The following section describes the effective use of this process in forming a partnership between decision makers and pharmacists to address a critical issue in long-term care.

Many aspects of long-term care pharmacy practice are different from traditional community practice because of the unique prescriber–patient–pharmacist relationships within a skilled-nursing facility (SNF). These differences often are not recognized by pharmacy regulators, since their experiences are usually with community pharmacy. One issue is that in SNFs, patient prescription orders are a part of the medical chart. The nurse must communicate with the physician and the pharmacy when the patient has medication needs. Since the facility nurse cannot take orders directly from the pharmacist, the nurse acts as a conduit between the pharmacy and the physician.

Many state boards of pharmacy are not sufficiently familiar with this process and thus have not drafted practice standards addressing it. Pharmacists in the LTC setting decided that this and other issues needed to be addressed by state boards of pharmacy nationwide. Working through their professional society, ASCP, a group of LTC pharmacists convened a task force that identified the issues as well as solutions that could be incorporated into state pharmacy practice acts. Rather than work independently in all 50 states, the group developed a strategy for working with the association that represents all 50 state boards (the National Association of Boards of Pharmacy, NABP) to alert regulators to these problems and request participation in the development of solutions.

The result was a cooperative effort between these pharmacists and NABP to develop model regulations governing the practice of LTC pharmacy that would be included in NABP's model pharmacy practice act. NABP's model practice act language serves as a national standard and provides pharmacists in each state common ground for working with their respective boards. This example shows how resources can be garnered within one's own group (here, a pharmacy professional society) and other related groups (NABP, in this case). This effort by LTC pharmacists and the boards of pharmacy provides a strong foundation for success, but pharmacists in each state must build on it by working with their state boards to put these ideas into their practice acts. Without advocacy at the individual state level, these ideas will remain a model rather than a reality.

Summary

We have examined the differences between state and federal regulatory and legislative agendas and cycles, as well as issues that transcend both the states and Congress. The examples illustrate the need for the pharmacy profession to remain vigilant at both the state and federal levels. The trade groups and professional societies that represent pharmacy have a significant advocacy role. Key individuals in these organizations at both the state and national levels need to constantly monitor activity that may influence pharmacy practice. They must alert and mobilize members when the circumstances demand their involvement. Grassroots action is crucial for achieving the desired results.

Finally, we have outlined the importance of garnering resources and identifying other stakeholders to reinforce advocacy efforts. There is strength in numbers. When those advocating an issue join in a broad-based coalition, whether of pharmacy groups representing all practice settings or of additional interested groups, their case is stronger and more compelling. To protect our professional interests, pharmacists need to actively participate in ongoing advocacy that bridges the gap between national and state issues.

CHAPTER

APPLICATION OF ADVOCACY AND LEADERSHIP

Richard P. Penna

T he public expresses its will in a variety of ways. In our representative form of government, legislation and regulation are means of expressing the voice of the people. Professions, speaking and acting through their professional societies, attempt to promote their goals and objectives by passing legislation or supporting the adoption of regulations.

Professional organizations' strategies for achieving their legislative and regulatory goals include political or legislative advocacy, lobbying, and public relations. Each of these strategies has advantages and disadvantages. The wise pharmacy leader understands the differences between these strategies and chooses the one that will be most effective and have the fewest disadvantages.

This chapter discusses advocacy, lobbying, and public relations as potential strategies for individual practitioners and their professional associations. It outlines the strengths and weaknesses of each, and it uses personal experiences to illustrate. Following each topic, the key point, or "lesson learned," appears in italic type.

Richard P. Penna

Background

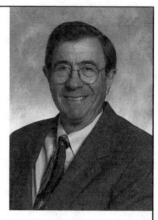

Richard Penna graduated with a bachelor of science in pharmacy in 1958 and PharmD in 1959 from the University of California, San Francisco. He was a community pharmacist in Redwood City, California, from 1959 to 1966 and assistant clinical professor at his alma mater from 1961 to 1966. He served as Peninsula Pharmaceutical Society president in 1960–61, San Mateo Pharmaceutical Association president in 1965–66, and *California Pharmacy* pharmaceutical editor in 1964–66. He joined the staff of the American Pharmaceutical Association (APhA) in 1966, serving as executive secretary of the Academy of General Practice of Pharmacy from 1966 through 1973, director of professional affairs from 1973 through 1983, director of the APhA *Handbook of Nonprescription Drugs* from 1975 through 1980, secretary of the Board of Pharmaceutical Specialties from 1976 through 1983, and vice president for professional affairs and Academy of Pharmacy Practice executive secretary in 1983–84. He also served on the National Health Council board of directors from 1973 through 1980 and as vice president from 1977 through 1980.

Penna joined the staff of the American Association of Colleges of Pharmacy (AACP) in 1985, serving as associate executive director from 1985 through 1995 and executive vice president from 1995 through 2002. He also served as Federation of Associations of Schools of the Health Professions treasurer from 1998 through 2002. During his tenure at AACP, he helped reshape pharmacy education to meet the changing needs of the profession.

He is a recipient of the Remington Honor Medal, pharmacy's highest honor.

Advocacy

Advocacy is a broad term covering a variety of activities used by individuals and professional societies to persuade the public or its elected representatives to do something that the profession deems beneficial. The verb "to advocate" encompasses the many actions used to promote a policy position. The most effective form of advocacy is the daily activities of individual practitioners as they serve the needs of clients or patients seeking their advice, counsel, diagnosis, treatment, or care. Indeed, the most skillfully crafted lobbying or public relations campaign will fail and even backfire if it is not supported by the experiences of the public and its representatives in dealing with their own health care practitioners.

I once was on the staff of the American Pharmaceutical Association (APhA; now the American Pharmacists Association) and editor of several early editions of the APhA *Handbook of Nonprescription Drugs*. Because of my position, I was often consulted by members of the press about nonprescription medications. One consumer writer called frequently with questions related to nonprescription products or product classes. Each time, I suggested that, in his column, the writer should encourage readers to ask their pharmacists about what specific products to use, but he did not take my suggestion. Then one day he called to tell me what had happened when he had gone to a pharmacy for a nonprescription cold remedy. Because of a prescription medication the writer was taking, the pharmacist had advised him against the cold remedy that he had heard advertised and was about to purchase. The writer was so impressed that he wrote a nationally distributed column on the value of consulting pharmacists on medication-related questions. Not only had the pharmacist fulfilled her professional responsibility to a patient, but she had performed a valuable act of advocacy for her profession.

Another example occurred when I was visiting a state legislator about an important pharmacy bill before the state assembly. The legislator listened intently and politely to my presentation. When I finished and asked if she had any questions, she proceeded to tell me about a recent experience at her local pharmacy. She had had a prescription renewed, but the tablets were a different color and shape from what she had been receiving. When she questioned the pharmacist about the discrepancy, the pharmacist reacted defensively and abusively. She was made to feel very uncomfortable, as if the problem had been her fault. She asked me if this was the type of professional that we were producing in our schools. That pharmacist, regardless of the reasons that may have caused his unprofessional outburst, did incalculable harm to the advocacy efforts of his profession.

A key point in both of these examples is that the pharmacists were not aware that their professional or unprofessional acts had served an advocacy function. The message for all pharmacists and pharmacy leaders is that, at any time, the services you render may have critical downstream impact on the public's view of our profession.

The Basis of Advocacy

The profession's policy (that is, what it advocates), whether formulated and adopted by local, state, or national organizations, needs to be consistent with the public good. If the public cannot see a benefit for itself in the policy, it will not support it. Moreover, policy that is expressed in terms of economic benefit for the profession will be viewed as self-serving. Health professions are dedicated to improving the public health; all aspects of a health professional organization's policies must be directed toward maximizing the profession's contributions to the health and well-being of the public.

The effective pharmacy leader is sensitive to the profession's obligation to the public and ensures that the profession's positions are expressed in terms that support the public good.

Policy Means What to Advocate

This may seem obvious, but an effective advocacy program must begin with a clear idea of what the individual or organization wishes to achieve. This idea is usually described as "policy," a term that is frequently misunderstood. Achieving consensus within an organization as to what its advocacy goals should be is no easy task. Still more daunting is stating the policy in concise, understandable, and persuasive language. In the context of advocacy, however, policy means simply a description of the organization's or society's desired outcomes, stated clearly and unambiguously so that all who read or hear it will understand what is desired and why.

A major responsibility of leadership and individual leaders is understanding the importance of clarity and the need for consensus within the organization. A leader who believes that he or she knows what is needed and proceeds to craft advocacy language without the participation and input of the membership is courting disaster. The debate that accompanies the development of policy helps clarify the language of and underlying reasons for the proposed policy. The effective leader will stimulate debate and discussion; he or she will listen carefully to all points of view and craft final language that includes all relevant perspectives. Thus, the person who drafts the policy statement has the most critical position in the policy development process.

The effective pharmacy leader understands the importance of drafting clear statements of policy and often performs that role.

Terminology Is Important

Words mean different things to different people. In preparing policy statements, leaders must take great care to select and use terminology that best conveys the intended ideas, in a light that reflects well on the policy and the organization promoting it. Generally, policy statements are expressed in positive rather than negative terms. A specific position may be a negative one (e.g., to oppose a legislative initiative or regulatory proposal), but it should stem from a positive policy position based on the profession's support of the public good. The following examples underscore the need for careful word choice.

In the 1970s APhA embarked on a policy initiative that would grant to pharmacists the professional right to select and dispense a generic product equivalent to one prescribed by brand name. Opponents of the policy called it "substitution," a pejorative term that put proponents on the defensive immediately. APhA leadership countered with the term "drug product selection," which placed the focus on a legitimate professional act of pharmacists in fulfilling their responsibility to patients to dispense quality drug products at reasonable costs.

Another example occurred a few years later when APhA was considering a policy advocating that pharmacists in organized health systems dispense drug products that were therapeutically equivalent to the one prescribed. Opponents jumped on this policy as "therapeutic substitution," whereas APhA established the term "therapeutic interchange." Other terms, such as "protocol prescribing" and "collaborative prescribing," subsequently have come into fashion to describe this important professional function.

Leaders who contemplate developing policy positions in areas where opposition is already forming would do well to study the terminology used by opponents and adopt other terminology. Words that opponents use do not necessarily put pharmacy in a good light.

Even in areas where little or no opposition exists, terminology must be carefully chosen to convey information accurately. A case in point is the entry-level degree that colleges and schools of pharmacy award. Many of our leaders mistakenly refer to the Doctor of Pharmacy degree as the "6-year PharmD." This is an inaccurate description of the degree; it conveys the impression to the uninitiated that pharmacists receiving the degree have gone to school (college) for 6 years after high school. In fact, most pharmacy colleges and schools offer a program that is 4 academic years in length, but a majority of students who enter pharmacy school have 3 or more years of college beforehand. In length and format of the curriculum, pharmaceutical education is similar to medical and dental education.

Referring to pharmacy education as a 6-year program, when a small minority of schools offer a PharmD degree in 6 years, conveys misinformation to the public.

Influencing Legislation and Regulation

Pharmacy leaders often must take their policy positions to local, state, or federal governments to secure legislation or regulation to implement the policies. Organized pharmacy has played an important role in efforts to maintain individual practitioners' freedom to practice as well as to expand the profession's scope of practice through legislative or regulatory actions. National and state pharmacy associations expend considerable resources supporting their legislative advocacy. The effective pharmacy leader ensures that professional policies are not only directed to the public good but are also clearly written and articulately and aggressively presented. There are two principal methods of influencing legislation and regulation: lobbying and individual actions.

Lobbying.   Lobbying is a form of advocacy in which one person or an organization attempts to influence the legislative process (either supporting or opposing legislation) or the regulatory process (either supporting or opposing proposed regulations) through direct visits with legislators or regulators. For lobbying visits to be effective, they must be supported by appropriate policy statements and other information bolstering the position being advocated.

Professional societies and organizations may choose to carry out the lobbying function themselves by supplying the policy statements and personnel, or they may hire a lobbying firm. Both have advantages and disadvantages, despite the common misconception that all problems can be solved and all legislation enacted by hiring the right lobbying firm and paying enough. Lobbying firms often retain individuals who previously served as elected legislators or members of a legislator's staff. These individuals have an intimate understanding of the legislative process. It is not uncommon for them to know legislators and legislative staff personally. It is important to understand that although lobbying firms may facilitate contact with legislators and regulators, they cannot develop policy positions. They may assist in the crafting of a statement, but the policy must come from the profession. Furthermore, a lobbying organization is most effective when individual practitioners (especially constituents of the intended legislator) make the visits. Finally, lobbying firms are expensive. The decision to hire such a firm must be based on an analysis of financial resources, the availability of dedicated practitioners to work with the firm, and the value of the anticipated legislative or regulatory gain to the profession.

Individual actions.   The late Congressman Thomas "Tip" O'Neill said, "All politics is local." Successful efforts to influence legislation are based on the relationship that exists between individual practitioners and their legislator. Efforts to influence legislation and regulation must be grounded in a clear understanding of the profession for which regulations are being drafted. Even if a professional society hires a lobbying firm, it will insist on individual practitioners being involved in legislative visits.

Most national and state pharmacy associations sponsor legislative days or conferences in which members gather for briefings and visits to their legislators. As noted in Chapter 7, these are valuable exercises, but they do not take the place of long-term relationships between individual practitioners and their elected representatives. These relationships are built on frequent visits while the legislator is in his or her home district and support at election time. The latter may take the form of making financial contributions, hosting campaign fundraising events, or being a volunteer who works in the campaign office, distributes literature, or performs other activities. Personal visits while the legislator is in the home district have advantages over visits to the state or national capital. While at home, legislators are not as busy as during the legislative session. In home district visits there is time to discuss a variety of issues. Legislators often ask for opinions on issues unrelated to pharmacy and drug policy, just to learn more about what their constituents are thinking. The following two examples illustrate this.

> *The effective pharmacy leader ensures that professional policies are not only directed to the public good but are also clearly written and articulately and aggressively presented.*

When the Department of Health, Education, and Welfare (precursor of the Department of Health and Human Services) was writing regulations to support the newly adopted Medicare bill, it asked a Public Health Service pharmacist to draft regulations covering the use of medications in nursing homes. Because that pharmacist was intimately familiar with the need for professional oversight of medication use in organized health care facilities, he wrote into the regulations that all medications used in Medicare patients cared for in nursing homes must be reviewed monthly by a consultant pharmacist. The regulation was adopted, and there sprang up a new professional area in pharmacy, that of consulting pharmacy, and a new professional society to support the educational and professional needs of pharmacists who began providing services to nursing home patients.

In another example, a pharmacy school dean was visiting his Senator on Capitol Hill. The dean had developed a long and close relationship with his Senator, had supported him in his home state, and had frequently met with him in his local and Washington offices. At the time of the visit, the Senate was considering legislation to support health professions education and thereby increase the supply of all health professionals to meet the growing demand caused by the recently enacted Medicare program. The Senator was chair of the committee responsible for developing the legislation, and the Senator asked the dean, while he was in the office, to write down some important points that should be in the pharmaceutical education part of the larger bill. The dean did, and in so doing he wrote that segment of the bill. As it happened, clinical pharmacy had recently been articulated as a new and very popular expansion of pharmacy practice. The dean wrote into the bill that in order for any pharmacy school to receive funds under the act, it must teach clinical pharmacy as part of its curriculum. Those few sentences in a funding bill were responsible for the rapid expansion of clinical pharmacy education.

The effective pharmacy leader is aware of a variety of current legislative issues and can articulate informed and intelligent views.

Support versus Championing

There is a difference between supporting a legislative effort and championing it. Both are important, but it is critical to recognize the difference. A legislator may indicate support for a constituent's view on a legislative matter, but many constituents may visit the legislator to express conflicting positions on a particular bill. Therefore, a legislator who indicates support for a bill or amendment may vote either for or against it. When the bill comes up for a vote in committee or on the floor, the legislator will have to weigh all of the constituents' positions.

In contrast, championing a position means that the legislator will introduce a bill or amendment, aggressively pursue its adoption, seek support of other legislators, and take whatever action is necessary to secure its passage. Every legislative action requires one or more champions; the more there are, the better. Champions are needed not only to pass a bill but to successfully oppose legislation. The difference between support and championing is the amount of energy expended. In most cases, champions expend "political capital" as well; this means asking for the support of colleagues in return for past political favors.

The effective pharmacy leader understands that not every legislator is able to or wants to be a champion of a legislative position. A legislator who is in the political minority may not be able or willing to "stick his/her neck out" on an issue. The legislator may already be championing too much legislation. Or the legislator may not feel sufficiently excited about the position to want to expend energy and political capital pursuing it. The pharmacy leader must recognize these possibilities, thank the legislator, and continue to seek his or her support in the future. The legislator may suggest others who would be more willing or more effective champions.

Pharmacy leaders who consistently and frequently visit and support their representatives will find it easier to enlist their support as champions.

Keep At It

Legislative advocacy is not an activity to be pursued on an annual or periodic basis. To be successful, advocacy requires consistent effort and attention. Just as a flower garden requires constant maintenance to produce beautiful blooms, a pharmacy leader's legislative "garden" needs constant nurturing. Beneficial results may come unexpectedly and in ways not imagined, as in the following example.

I spend considerable time in the state legislature advocating for pharmacy's needs. A state senator in the district adjoining mine occupied a key committee position even though he was a member of the minority political party. I called him to ask that he support our position on a particular issue. This was during the legislative session, and I could not get an appointment with him in time. He said that students had visited him and he had been persuaded to support our position. After the session concluded, I went to his district office to thank him for his support. (Always thank your legislator!) Since growing wine grapes and making wine is one of my hobbies, I took him a bottle of my wine as a thank-you gift. This led us into a discussion of wine grape growing in our area. I was also active in my state wine grape growers association, and we had been pursuing legislation supporting the expansion of the grape and wine industry in our state. This legislator from an agricultural district was very concerned about the declining incomes from milk and apple production in his district. As a result of our discussion, he called a meeting of the state secretary of agriculture and other top agriculture officials. As a result of that meeting, the secretary of agriculture asked the governor to appoint a task force to consider issues related to expanding wine grape growing and wineries in our state. I was appointed to that task force and made its chair. Our report, issued 3 months later, was the basis of several successful pieces of legislation introduced by this senator and adopted by the state legislature.

This senator could not be a champion of pharmacy legislation, although he supported it, but he became a strong champion of the wine industry in our state. Someday, under different political circumstances, he may become a champion of pharmacy legislation. Although we are of different political parties, I will support his re-election financially and in whatever way he may request. Some would say our meeting was serendipitous. In this case, the results benefited my state's wine industry. In a subsequent session of the legislature, this senator was influential in a joint committee that approved planning funds for the state school of pharmacy building.

Being legislatively active over time is bound to produce beneficial results.

Media Relations

Media relations is an important part of advocacy. It could be considered as a part of public relations; however, public relations campaigns must be ongoing to be effective, and they can be extremely expensive. Media relations is smaller in scope than public relations and can be carried out by individual pharmacy leaders as well as pharmaceutical organizations. Media relations is the development and maintenance of close relations with specific members of the media, including print, radio, and television. Much of what the public reads, sees, and hears in the media related to health and medications is associated with the medical profession. It is important for the public to read, see, and hear that pharmacists possess comprehensive knowledge about medications and have the expertise to improve medication use. The effective pharmacy leader will cultivate relationships with members of the media. He or she will offer clear and informed commentary on issues or refer the media to those who will be able to respond with accurate information. Most often this begins with a pharmacist who renders competent, caring, and conspicuous service to all patients, including those who may be members of the media. It is difficult to explain to a television producer that pharmacists render valuable service if the producer's personal experience speaks to the contrary.

Like legislative relations, media relations take time to cultivate, but once established can be extremely beneficial to the profession.

Conclusion

Advocacy is a critical and necessary part of the pharmacy leader's role. Understanding the comprehensive nature of advocacy is the leader's first challenge. Advocacy involves understanding relevant policy issues; expressing them in clear language; understanding the processes of securing public, legislative, and regulatory support for policies; and engaging in the arduous process of securing adoption of pharmacy's positions.

Advocacy is a long-term effort that does not promise immediate results. It is also a personal act that frequently relies on close relationships. Advocacy is a leadership function. The person who does not advocate is not a leader.

USING PUBLIC RELATIONS TO ADVOCATE FOR THE PROFESSION

David A. Holdford

I f you spend any time watching television, surfing the Internet, listening to the radio, or reading newspapers and magazines, you have been touched by public relations campaigns. In truth, most of us are pretty savvy about public relations because we have been bombarded by those campaign messages continually throughout our lives. We have been exposed to causes ranging from the American Cancer Society's campaign to fund cancer research to the federal government's crusade against drug and alcohol abuse. The pharmacy profession has been engaged in its own public relations campaign over the years—for greater responsibility and recognition of the important role of proper medication use in patient health. This chapter provides tools and guidance for using public relations to get pharmacy's message out to our "publics"—the audiences with whom we want to communicate.

I first became interested in public relations when I was chair of a local chapter of the Sierra Club, an environmental advocacy organization. Our group in Columbia, South Carolina, had more

See author profile on page 28.

than 1,000 members involved in promoting energy conservation, controlling water and air pollution, preserving wildlife and lands, and advocating for other environmental causes. The club's mission was to support environmental legislation, educate the public, and provide opportunities to become involved in protecting the environment. Success in recruiting, fundraising, and lobbying depended greatly on our positive relations with the general public.

My introduction to lobbying and advocating legislative changes concerned a state energy legislation initiative that was charged with proposing new laws affecting energy use. Because our local Sierra Club chapter had developed extensive contacts in the statehouse over the years and had good relations within the community, we were invited to send representatives to sit on several task forces proposing energy conservation laws. Without the foundation of the relationships and goodwill the group had developed previously with public and government representatives, we would never have had the opportunity to influence laws affecting the environment. We were able to have several of our initiatives included in the legislation that was enacted.

Public relations is equally important for promoting the causes supported by pharmacists. The success of organized advocacy for the pharmacy profession depends greatly on collective goodwill developed by pharmacists and pharmacy organizations over time. The goodwill of patients, health care professionals, and others is a valuable asset founded on the strength and quality of relationships we have with the public. As discussed in previous chapters, pharmacists who develop strong, positive relationships can use those networks to influence change.

Public relations is defined as the process of building relationships between an entity and its publics. In pharmacy, it deals with the way pharmacists interact with and are perceived by important audiences that range from patients to funding agencies. Successful public relations creates a climate in the community supportive of the goals and programs of pharmacy practice. Its purpose is to establish a favorable, informed image in the minds of the public about pharmacists and the profession.

Public relations encompasses a broad range of activities that enhance our professional image. It is sometimes confused with publicity, which refers to organized efforts to manage the spread of information about an issue or product. Publicity is just one element of public relations. Public relations activities include the following:[1]

- Lobbying—advocating for a cause with legislatures and government agencies
- Government relations—communicating with and educating legislatures and government agencies
- Media relations—dealing with the media in seeking publicity or stimulating interest for a cause
- Publicity—communicating with the public through media (e.g., press releases, news conferences)
- Direct communications with constituents
- Public appearances before groups, such as speeches or seminars (Figure 14-1 lists steps for conducting media events)
- Community relations—dealing with citizens and groups within an area

All of these overlapping activities help create a strong favorable impression with the public and gain support for our cause.

✓ Call your first meeting.
✓ Choose a chair and members of the planning committee.
✓ Identify goals and objectives for the event
  (e.g., how will you know if you are successful?).
✓ List necessary tasks and assign responsibility.
✓ Identify a site for the event and request permission to use the site.
✓ Develop a plan to promote the event.
✓ Make a budget and identify sources of funding for the event
  (e.g., sponsors).
✓ Map out a timeline for tasks. Schedule future meetings.
✓ At least 1 week before the event: Confirm the room, speakers, and
  refreshments. Review responsibilities of participants and confirm the
  number of attendees. Personally contact any "VIPs" whose attendance you
  especially want.
✓ On the day of the event: Distribute a schedule or agenda to committee
  members, review assignments, and answer questions. Confirm room
  readiness, audiovisual equipment, and speakers.
✓ After the event, send thank-you letters to speakers and committee
  members.
✓ Write and send out a press release or other promotional announcement.
✓ Conduct a postevent assessment.

FIGURE 14-1   Sample Media Event Checklist

Advantages and Disadvantages of Public Relations

The primary advantage of public relations is that it can help you get your message across without spending much money. Although it is possible to spend thousands of dollars on large public relations campaigns, it is feasible to inexpensively promote your cause through press coverage and member lobbying of public officials. An additional advantage is that public relations can build credibility. Messages promoted through news coverage, editorials, and endorsements from public officials are viewed more favorably than advertising and other types of paid promotional communications.[2]

The downside of public relations is that it can be ignored or distorted. Third parties, such as editors and public officials, have no obligation to pick up and promote your ideas. They may not see you as newsworthy or important. Even worse, they may distort your message in an undesirable way. An unscrupulous reporter can twist a television press interview meant to promote professional pharmacist services into a sensationalistic exposé on pharmacist errors. The key to avoiding such situations is to master the art of public relations.

Building Strong Professional Relationships

Public relations builds strong relationships between pharmacist advocates and their target audiences by managing "professional goodwill." Goodwill toward the pharmacy profession is based on the positive images and associations that come to mind when people hear the words "pharmacy" or "pharmacist." Goodwill can be associated with individuals (e.g., Mary, the pharmacist), organizations (e.g., our national professional pharmacy organizations), ideas (e.g., medication therapy management services), and any other entity for which one advocates. Public relations attempts to influence perceptions so that the public will back our profession.

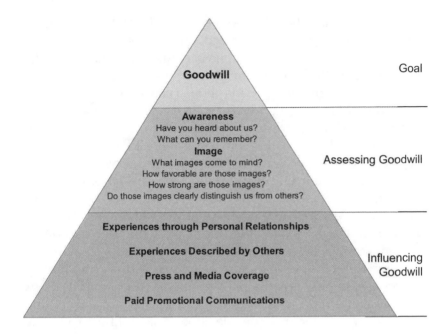

FIGURE 14-2   Building Goodwill

Goodwill comes from a mix of mental associations with what is being advocated. Goodwill toward "pharmacists" depends on public images that may be positive (e.g., trustworthy), negative (e.g., a pill counter), or nonexistent. Advocates attempt to build an image where there is none, strengthen positive images that already exist, and repair negative images. Figure 14-2 depicts how goodwill is assessed and factors that influence it.

Assessing Goodwill

Goodwill is a function of the public's awareness of a cause. The strength of public perceptions is determined by the extent that people recognize a cause when they see it and recall it when prompted. Familiarity is a prerequisite for public support. Goodwill also depends on the dominant image that members of the public associate with their awareness of a cause—the image that immediately comes to mind upon hearing about your cause. In marketing, this is called "brand meaning." Ideally, images associated with your cause should accurately depict what you are trying to achieve. To arouse public backing, they should also be favorable, strongly formed, and distinct.

Awareness of and perceptions about a cause come from a variety of sources. The most powerful sources are direct and indirect experiences. Disease advocacy groups like the American Cancer Society understand this when they solicit cancer survivors and their friends and family members to participate in activities such as the Relay for Life. People who have directly or indirectly experienced the disease are the most fervent advocates of funding for cancer research and other American Cancer Society goals. Coverage in the press and other forms of media is an additional source of knowledge about advocacy causes. Media sources that are perceived to be credible, such as Oprah Winfrey, can greatly influence opinions. Finally, paid promotional communications such as television, radio, Internet, and newspaper advertising help inform and persuade people about causes. Effective public relations attempts to influence all of these sources.

Developing a Public Relations Plan

Effective public relations starts with a well thought out strategic plan. It involves defining what you want to achieve, identifying the target audience you wish to influence, developing and delivering a clear message, and assessing your success. The plan should outline what will be done, by whom, and by when. Steps typically follow a timeline for accomplishing tasks to encourage progression toward your final objective.

Step 1: Define your objective. Public relations objectives should originate from and complement your overall mission. Otherwise, you will be wasting your effort on things that are not important. Good objectives should be measurable so that you can quantify your success. An example of a public relations objective for promoting an important event might be "Achieve attendance of at least 100 people." If at least that many people attend, you know you were successful.

Objectives should be focused and not overly ambitious. It is better to do a few tasks well than many tasks poorly. Focus ensures continued credibility with the public and a greater likelihood of success. That success, in turn, often attracts new recruits to your cause and further support from target audiences. People love success, so it is easier to build on a few accomplishments than a mixed track record of successes and failures.

Step 2: Know your audience. Every organization has publics whose opinions and assistance are important. The pharmacy profession's publics include patients, pharmacists, employers, funding agencies, other health professionals, politicians, and pharmaceutical companies. The needs of each public vary, and the messages directed at them should too.

The more you know about your publics, the better you can craft a message that will reach them and spark their interest. Public information sources (e.g., a politician's personal Web site) can be useful for learning about official viewpoints on issues, but the best way to learn is to engage in conversation. If you care about influencing legislation, you should speak to a politician or someone on the politician's staff. If you want to influence media coverage, you should talk to reporters and editors. You may be surprised how welcoming these individuals can be. They are people doing their jobs like everyone else, and they often need you as much as you need them. The media need interesting stories and people who can relate them in an engaging way, and politicians must understand the perspectives of constituents in order to gain their backing. Be aware that you have a lot to offer.

There are two phases of communication with your publics. The first is an information gathering stage that introduces you to each other and identifies mutual perspectives and needs. Personal visits are ideal, but busy schedules do not always permit them. Telephone and e-mail are also good choices. The key is to develop a relationship with your publics prior to the time you need them. The second phase consists of approaching them with your message, through the media or other form of communication. If you have learned about their interests and preferences beforehand, you can tailor a message that will please you both. Table 14-1 contains suggestions for communicating with media representatives.

TABLE 14-1 Approaching the Media

Know the decision makers. Don't waste your time or any one else's by speaking with the wrong people. Look through media directories on the Web or in the library to find the names, addresses, and phone numbers of health editors, reporters, and assignment editors.

Know your story. Know what you will say and how you are going to say it. Rehearse it so it will flow well. Know the guidelines for reporting stories such as yours.

Choose the medium. Be certain that your story is right for the medium you approach.

Respect others' time and deadlines. A missed deadline destroys credibility for you and pharmacy advocates who follow. Always keep your promises and respect all deadlines. Be prepared.

Be polite but persistent. Do not be discouraged if the local media do not run your story the first time you approach them. If they have to change their plans at the last moment, reschedule a new time. If problems occur, suggest solutions. Be assertive and flexible in suggesting new ideas, but do not press your cause too hard. Make it easy for the media to use your stories.

Adapted from reference 1.

Step 3: Craft your message. You may have an important message for the public, but it may never be heard if you do not say it well and concisely. What you say and how you say it will determine your effectiveness. Use positive language that conveys a proactive message, rather than a reactive one. For example, a report on medication errors could be more positively presented as best practices for error prevention. When advocating for our profession, you may want to work some of the following themes[1] into your messages.

- Pharmacy has expanded its role within health care from a profession focusing on preparing and dispensing medications to one emphasizing a wide range of patient-oriented services designed to maximize the effectiveness of medicines.
- Pharmacy is practiced in a broad range of settings: independent and chain community pharmacies, hospitals, long-term care facilities, the pharmaceutical industry, mail service, academia, managed care, and government.
- Medications have the power to heal when taken correctly but can cause serious harm when used inappropriately. The pharmacist's role is to help patients achieve the benefits of drugs and avoid harm.

- Pharmacists have extensive education about drugs and the diseases that they treat. They are the best health professional to assist patients with their medications.
- Patients should choose a pharmacist they trust and develop a partnership for good health. A pharmacist who knows you and your health needs can best help you prevent harmful drug interactions, avoid allergic reactions, save money on your drugs, and take drugs in the most effective manner.

After choosing what to say, you must deliver the message in a manner that presents these benefits in a meaningful way. Storytelling is a powerful tool for building meaning through situations or examples. Public relations messages, then, should be designed from the audience's perspective and should consider the following:[1]

- Will your message be of interest to members of the public? Does it appeal to things they consider important? Is it told in an engaging, entertaining way?
- How does your message match up against competing messages? Would it compare favorably with stories seen in magazines, newspapers, or electronic media?
- Is your message timely? Look for an element that makes it appropriate for immediate release.
- What outcome do you want to achieve with your message? Are you attempting to inform, persuade, or remind your audience?
- Whom are you attempting to reach? Is your message crafted in a way that your target audience can understand and appreciate?
- Is your message simple and easy to comprehend? Is it memorable?

Step 4: Multiply your message.   Good public relations messages can build on each other. A single article or idea in the media can have a snowball effect when it is picked up and passed on by various media sources and key opinion leaders. The chance that this will occur depends in part on luck, but the likelihood increases if you identify and maintain contact with the right individuals and media sources and use multiple means of communication to increase opportunities for audiences to hear a message.

You can help your messages to snowball by publicizing the publicity you receive. If a newspaper article is published about your cause, you can send a press release to a radio station or magazine summarizing the newspaper article. If a member of your organization receives an award or does something of note, it can be publicized in a letter to the editor or a media alert. The following basic public relations tools can be used to publicize your activities:

- Pitch letters. A pitch letter introduces you to an editor, producer, or other key individual. The pitch letter is used as an initial step to setting up a personal interview, suggesting media stories, and obtaining media coverage.
- Press releases. A press (or news) release is a document issued to the media informing them about an event, idea, story, or other newsworthy item. It is typically directed at journalists and editors of media organizations with the hope that the information will generate a positive media story or mention.
- Media kits. A media kit is a folder containing print materials to inform interested media representatives about your organization, its activities, and its goals. The media kit can contain any relevant material that you want to communicate about your organization.
- Letters to the editor. These letters are designed to promote some issue on the editorial pages of print media. They help communicate your message and can help establish you as an expert on a given topic.
- Media advisories or alerts. These draw attention to an event that you want the media to attend and cover. They contain the who, what, when, where, why, and how of the event. They are typically sent to the media 1 or 2 days before the event.
- Feature articles. The media will print human interest stories that may promote your cause. If the theme and angle of the article are appealing, you may be asked to supply background information to a reporter or to even write the article yourself.
- Op-eds. Op-eds are articles expressing opinions and typically published on editorial pages of newspapers. They may be solicited if you are a recognized expert or accepted when submitted "cold" if they are timely and well written.

TABLE 14-2   Conducting Radio and TV Interviews

Be prepared. Know your objectives and practice your responses to questions. If you have not received a list of questions that will be covered, ask for one. If you are being interviewed on television or radio, you do not want to be grasping for the best way to phrase a difficult issue. Craft your message in an interesting way that will be remembered positively. Anticipate questions and prepare responses.

Speak at your own pace. Do not feel the need to rush. Take time to listen to the question, think, and answer. Do not stray from your areas of expertise. Do not let your responses ramble.

Drive the interview. The media representative will ask the questions, but you can control the interview by how you answer them. Sometimes you may need to rephrase questions in a way that makes sense to you. Tactfully correct any errors or misstatements of fact.

Stay on your talking points. Continue to answer questions in a way that brings the interview back to points you want to emphasize. Take every opportunity to reemphasize your points.

Emphasize key words and phrases. Use the word "pharmacist" often in your sentences ("Pharmacists are experts in…" or "As a pharmacist, I always…"). If you have a slogan or sound bite to emphasize (e.g., pharmacists are medication experts), try to say it at the beginning, middle, and end of the interview.

Be engaging. Show enthusiasm for your topic. Speak up, and don't forget to smile. Emphasize positive information. Use interesting stories and anecdotes to illustrate your points. Maintain eye contact, and use the interviewer's name.

Adapted from reference 1.

- Public service announcements (PSAs). PSAs are brief messages of helpful information provided to the public in print, audio, or video formats. They are carried free of charge by media organizations to educate audiences and promote causes.
- Broadcast interviews. Radio and TV interviews can promote your message powerfully to large populations. Tips for conducting broadcast interviews are provided in Table 14-2.

For examples of public relations tools and directions on their use, go to the American Pharmacists Association Web site (www.aphanet.org).

Step 5: Measure the result. If you have defined a quantifiable measure of success, assessing the impact of your public relations plan is straightforward. You may consider yourself successful if you get interviewed on the news, publish a letter to the editor, or conduct several legislative visits with members of your organization. You should share the successes with other advocates, and your results should be used to inform your future actions.

Responding to Emergencies

The role of public relations is not only to promote good news but also to positively influence bad news. Public relations emergencies can seriously damage the integrity of pharmacists if handled poorly. At the same time, emergencies can be an opportunity to highlight some of the profession's themes by spotlighting our roles as medication experts. Disasters publicized in the media might include unethical behavior by individual pharmacists, controversies over pharmacy policies and practices, and incidents where a pharmacist's action or inaction resulted in patient harm.

Any crisis that threatens the image or reputation of pharmacists should be dealt with in a careful, organized, and timely manner with the goal of minimizing damage to goodwill. In any crisis, the best advice is to respond honestly and quickly. Key individuals in the organization affected should meet to craft a factual, truthful response that recognizes the seriousness of the problem. Ideally, responses should come from a limited number of individuals to ensure a consistent, accurate message. Spokespeople should be the most eloquent and competent public speakers available. Student pharmacists can be excellent, credible spokespersons for many circumstances, but they should have some experience and training before responding to crises. Emergencies are not the ideal time for novice spokespeople to be speaking for the profession.

If you are known by the media and have experience interviewing, you may be asked to speak to them. Before you do, ask yourself if you are the right person to be interviewing. If not, forward inquiries to others who are more appropriate. If you feel that you can adequately address fast-breaking controversies, however, prepare what you are going to say. Because of the risks associated with making things worse, think carefully before you provide offhand comments. Stick with facts only, avoid blaming others, and try not to be defensive. Do not make excuses or deny the existence of a problem. Listen to the interviewer's questions and do not be rushed to respond quickly. And if you don't know the answer to a question, say so. Plan transitions back to your key facts and pre-planned comments or talking points.

The success of organized advocacy for the pharmacy profession depends greatly on collective goodwill developed by pharmacists and pharmacy organizations over time.

Conclusion

Public relations in support of advocacy should be truthful and free of propaganda in order to maintain the public's trust. Advocacy is built on trust, and all efforts should be aimed at projecting an image of honesty, openness, and public benefit. This chapter provides guidance on how pharmacists can use public relations to advocate for our causes. For an excellent and more detailed guide on public relations, read *Public Relations for Pharmacists* by Tina L. Pugliese.[1]

References

1. Pugliese TL. *Public Relations for Pharmacists*. 1st ed. Washington, DC: American Pharmaceutical Association; 2000.
2. Holdford DA. *Marketing for Pharmacists*. Washington, DC: American Pharmacists Association; 2003.

Epilogue: Next Steps

Robert S. Beardsley

Robert Pruitt, a professional facilitator and leadership development expert (www.robertpruitt.com), provided the following comments about his work with students at the University of Maryland School of Pharmacy.

Imagine a sunny day, temperature in the upper 70s, blue skies dotted with white, puffy clouds. Now, picture a small group of people standing in a circle holding hands on a grassy knoll. Sounds like a "We Are the World" moment, right? I'd been asked to participate in the first class meeting of the School of Pharmacy leadership class. My goal was to effectively communicate the message that vision (an ideal image of the future) is the foundation of leadership. Without a picture of where they want to go and what tomorrow could look like, whether leaders will make a difference is left to chance.

Standing outside the pharmacy building in plain sight of peers, staff, and strangers, and with building construction across the street, the students attempted to untangle themselves and form an open circle without letting go of one another's hands. They stepped over, under, and through each other's arms. Some provided possible solutions, a few said nothing, and others continuously pointed out the problems. The conversation switched back and forth between being problem focused and solution focused.

After 15 minutes, time was called and we discussed the students' experience. What I discovered was a group who had just moved beyond intellectualizing what leadership meant. They were living life in the moment with curiosity and focus. No longer simply in class, they were in a real-world, life-altering experience. This course was no longer about acquiring a grade. It was a charge to get clear about their natural ability to contribute and to choose to serve others with purpose.

Robert S. Beardsley

Personal Statement

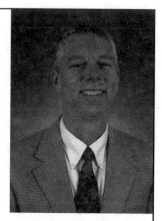

I have been involved with student leadership since my undergraduate years at Oregon State University (OSU), where I served as an officer in Rho Chi, Kappa Psi, and my social fraternity. My biggest challenge and opportunity during those years was serving as co-chair of the coordinating committee for Dads Weekend—planning activities for 15,000 students and their fathers. It was an exciting experience, and I enjoyed working with a variety of students, faculty, and administrators. Thanks to these and other efforts, I was selected for the Blue Key leadership honor society and was one of three in my graduating class to receive an Outstanding Leadership Award. I had several excellent mentors at OSU, and I agree with the messages in Chapter 5 about the importance of mentoring. In addition, I have been blessed with a wife, Kathy, who has also been involved with student activities during her professional career. The lessons that she and my mentors have taught me have been invaluable.

One lesson that I keep learning is how different people really are. They are motivated by different things, perceive the world differently than I do, and work differently under various leadership styles (as described in Chapter 3). As alluded to by several of this book's authors, effective leaders must pay attention to these differences as they work with others to fulfill the goals of their organizations. In the Effective Leadership and Advocacy course that I teach with my co-editors of this book, we discuss this point extensively. Students in the class cite many examples of times when they did not recognize these differences, and the faculty members have plenty of stories as well. Several years ago, I had the opportunity to facilitate the development of the Maryland Pharmacy Coalition, an organization formed by the major pharmacy associations in the state. During the process, I realized that each organization perceived pharmacy somewhat differently, had a different political agenda, and had a different idea about what the coalition should do. Fortunately, our planning group addressed these issues early so that we could eventually focus on the compelling reasons for the coalition's existence and the value of coming together.

In the 6 years that I've conducted leadership classes and retreats, I've watched students connect the vision concept and their vision statements (created as a small group activity) to their understanding of their organization's purpose. It's been great to witness this process. The vision-writing process provides student leaders with a gift—a conversation. Every leader must have something to say and share. These leadership experiences help remove haphazard behaviors and force these young leaders to take full responsibility for their relationships with staff and peers, the direction of their organizations, and the focus of their studies.

There are, however, challenges for these young leaders. One challenge is to constantly look beyond the walls of the school community and envision their potential impact on a larger scale. This means asking themselves difficult questions: How does my leadership affect the families in the surrounding neighborhoods? How does my vision translate to tangible results at the local, national, and global levels? How does an event hosted by my organization influence students, professors, staff, and community-based organizations? How can I live, each day, the mission of our school: education, research, and service? What are the rewards for living this mission? What are the costs? Am I helping to foster leadership in others? Am I a good follower?

Another challenge is to identify the weaknesses and strengths unique to student pharmacists. In general, I have observed weaknesses in those who are overly task oriented (analytical), reserved, slow to act, overcommitted, and quiet. But conversely, I have seen strengths among student pharmacists who are critical thinkers, problem solvers, task oriented, attentive to detail, passionate, and driven.

These challenges have value for teaching leadership and advocacy to tomorrow's professionals. Most of the students I've worked with express a need to make a contribution to our world. In pharmacy school they have found opportunities for leading change. Leadership requires that we advocate on behalf of those who cannot speak for themselves, and there are ample opportunities for this within and outside the school community. Within the school community there are students who never get involved in social action. They move from class to class and semester to semester thinking only of themselves. Sometimes, students feel small, swallowed up in the large student body, and think they have nothing to contribute. In many cases, students are waiting for someone—a leader—to extend a hand of fellowship.

Leadership also requires advocacy on behalf of other leaders who need support in times of great pressure or weakness. A few years ago, I conducted a leadership retreat for the school. A student leader—we'll call her Rebekah—had great responsibility as head of an on-campus organization. Her strength was in handling tasks. Her weakness was in fostering relationships, because she felt unable to speak up in large groups. During the retreat I issued Rebekah a leadership challenge: to stand in front of 40 of her peers and advisors and tell them what difference she wanted to make in the world. She reluctantly accepted my challenge. My advocacy began when she finished speaking. I continued asking questions and requiring impromptu responses. It was when she began to shake and cry that I knew she was facing her fear. I would not permit her to run from *the moment*, as was her habit. She cried and talked for the next 2 minutes, which for her seemed like a lifetime. Others in the room, inspired by her courage, began to verbally support her, as well as cry with her. A few wanted to rescue her from her experience. It was when Rebekah stood tall in the midst of her weakness that I stopped the activity, acknowledged her, and watched her dash out of the room. The room was uncomfortably silent. I was asked why I had put her through that activity. My response was that Rebekah put herself through that discovery process. It was clear that she was tired of running from that weakness. My advocacy role was to let her know she had the ability to share her thoughts in uncomfortable situations. When Rebekah returned to the room, everyone saw that she was still emotional but okay. The group, verbally and nonverbally, showed support for her. Some even hugged her. She said she'd never experienced anything like that before and was thankful for the activity. Even leaders need to be challenged in a way that supports growth through risk.

The preceding commentary illustrates an important point made by several authors in this textbook: To be an effective leader and advocate you must get out of your comfort zone—do something different, take a risk, feel uncomfortable in a new situation, as Rebekah did. For example, in Chapter 1, Dennis Worthen describes the contributions of key individuals in the profession who took risks and made a difference. Similarly, in Chapter 2, Lucinda Maine describes the contributions of pharmacy leaders (Donald Brodie and others) who saw the world differently and established their own path. The personal information provided by many of our contributing authors shows that they too took risks and went outside their comfort zone. For example, Arnie Clayman found himself to be the voice of long-term care pharmacy

in his state. As he put it, "It was a humbling experience and put me in situations beyond my comfort level, especially
when it came to legislative and political
issues. Until then, I had no great interest in these areas, but over time I grew
to understand the importance of being
involved in the process."

> *To be an effective leader and advocate you must get out of your comfort zone.*

Pruitt's comments also point out that
leaders must have a vision of where they want to go, as well as the
ability to share that vision with others in hope of securing their
support. Dennis Worthen illustrates this in Chapter 1 by describ-
ing the actions of numerous pharmacy leaders who crafted a
strong vision of what they wanted to accomplish and communicated it effectively to others. History reveals many situations
in which leaders have been successful, and other situations in
which success was compromised because leaders could not articulate their vision. For example, President Woodrow Wilson could
not convince an internally focused United States that the country
should support the League of Nations after World War I.

Although Pruitt's examples come from an academic setting,
the same leadership principles apply in pharmacy practice, to
seasoned pharmacists and new practitioners alike. John O'Brien's
comments in Chapter 6 clearly reveal the need for pharmacists
to develop strong leadership skills regardless of their practice
environment. In Chapter 3, David Holdford makes the point that
the principles in this book are based on documented leadership
theories and are not just random thoughts or ideas. Like Pruitt,
he stresses that leadership development must be anchored by a
strong theoretical framework.

Pruitt also speaks to the need for an organization and its
leaders to formulate a clear vision statement to guide the group
and set its priorities. Before preparing a vision statement, a
group must understand its purpose for existing. Several chapter authors support this point by noting that we should better
understand our roles, individually and collectively, as advocates
for pharmacy and for better patient care. In Chapter 7, Will Lang
describes possible roles within the federal legislative process,
and in Chapter 8 Theresa Wells Tolle discusses opportunities
for advocacy at the state level. In Chapter 10, Carriann Richey

discusses opportunities for using a professional lobbyist during our advocacy efforts. In order to understand our advocacy roles, we need to understand the legislative processes described by these authors. Furthermore, we must also understand the regulatory process in order to make an impact in this important area, and Ray Love provides guidance in Chapter 9 on where and how we can have the most influence on regulations.

In developing a vision, organizations must consider what values and issues are important to them. In Chapter 13 Richard Penna presents the important lessons that the values held by organizations should be reflected in their advocacy, lobbying, and public relations efforts, and that emerging policies must be focused on the public good. For our advocacy efforts to succeed, we must clearly articulate our values to legislators and regulators. Penna and other authors note that these value statements must be perceived as consistent and comprehensive throughout the organization.

In Chapter 11 Cynthia Boyle and Earlene Lipowski illustrate the potential influence of grassroots advocacy. They give practical suggestions and specific communication recommendations. Most important, they urge us to take just one step, one first step, toward active advocacy. The words of wisdom from pharmacist-legislator Bob Osterhaus ring true: "My best advice is to know who you are and why you believe what you do."

In closing, the editors would like to state that the success of this book will not be judged by how many copies are sold, but by what actions are taken by its readers. We acknowledge that learning about leadership and advocacy from sources such as this book is easy but implementing this knowledge may be difficult. It is relatively easy to state the essential attributes of an effective leader or advocate, and to recite suggested strategies for achieving success. The difficulty comes when you actually have to do it. The three of us remember how nervous we were when we made our first visit to our legislators, but now it seems as easy as giving a lecture to a group of pharmacists. (We still get nervous, but it is a controlled nervousness.) Unfortunately, for many of our colleagues, their first experiences at stepping outside their comfort zone were not positive. Thus, they were reluctant to try a second or third time. The key, as described by our authors, is to learn from our experiences, analyze the barriers and facilitators that we face, re-evaluate our strategies, and do it again. We wish you well with your future leadership and advocacy efforts.

INDEX

Note: Italic *t* refers to tables; italic *f* refers to figures.